Sex, Drugs, and HIV/AIDS in Brazil

W0234971

Sex, Drugs, and HIV/AIDS in Brazil

James A. Inciardi
Hilary L. Surratt
Paulo R. Telles

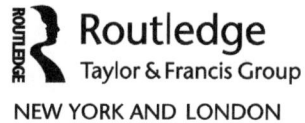

Routledge
Taylor & Francis Group

NEW YORK AND LONDON

First published 2000 by Westview Press

Published 2018 by Routledge
605 Third Avenue, New York, NY 10017
4 Park Square, Milton Park, Abingdon, Oxon OX14 4RN

Routledge is an imprint of the Taylor & Francis Group, an informa business

Copyright © 2000 Taylor & Francis

This research was supported by PHS Grant # UO1DAO–8510, "HIV/AIDS Community Outreach in Rio de Janeiro, Brazil," from the National Institute on Drug Abuse. The opinions expressed are those of the authors.

All rights reserved. No part of this book may be reprinted or reproduced or utilised in any form or by any electronic, mechanical, or other means, now known or hereafter invented, including photocopying and recording, or in any information storage or retrieval system, without permission in writing from the publishers.

Notice:
Product or corporate names may be trademarks or registered trademarks, and are used only for identification and explanation without intent to infringe.

Library of Congress Cataloging-in-Publication Data
Inciardi, James A.
    Favela and asfalto : sex, drugs, and HIV/AIDS in Brazil / James A. Inciardi, Hilary L. Surratt, Paulo R. Telles.
        p.   cm.
    Includes bibliographical references and index.
    ISBN 0-8133-3424-1 (pbk. : alk. paper)
    1. AIDS (Disease)—Brazil.   2. AIDS (Disease)—Brazil—Rio de Janeiro.   3. AIDS (Disease)—Brazil—Prevention.   4. AIDS (Disease)—Brazil—Rio de Janeiro—Prevention. 5. Urban poor—Health and hygiene—Brazil.   I. Surratt, Hilary L.   II. Telles, Paulo R.   III. Title

RA644.A25 I496   2000
362.1'969792'00981—dc21   00-043784

ISBN 13: 978-0-8133-3424-0 (pbk)

Contents

List of Tables and Illustrations

Preface

Since its settlement by the Portuguese in the 16th century, Brazil has provided ceaseless fascination for people in other parts of the world. Brazil has gold, rubber, and coffee. During and after World War II it was a place of refuge, and more recently it boasts the sights and sounds of the world's fifth largest nation. And then there are the Brazilians themselves, who enjoy one of the richest musical cultures in the world. Clearly the most sophisticated popular music across the globe, Brazilian "world beat" is a sensuous mélange of African, Indian, European, and American influences. Nightly in any major city, one can find internationally known jazz artists, regional musicians specializing in native rhythms, and both world-class and local dancers executing the complex moves of the bossa nova, *lambada*, *pagode*, and of course, the samba. And not to be forgotten is Antônio Carlos Jobim's "The Girl from Ipanema," considered by the music industry to be the most popular song ever recorded.

The geography of Brazil also is unique, diverse, and captivating. With the exception of Chile and Ecuador, Brazil borders every country in South America and occupies almost half the continent. There are the coastal mountain ranges, the vast wetlands of the Pantanal, and the lush Amazon basin and rain forest.

But despite its beauty and richness, Brazil faces many problems. For example, the country experiences major environmental challenges, which place much of its vast natural wealth under continuous threat. There is pollution and poaching in the Pantanal, where upwards of two million animals are killed each year. There is the exploitation and destruction of the Amazon. This large, complex, and fragile ecosystem—comprising one-tenth of the Earth's plant and animal species, producing one-fifth of the world's oxygen, and containing one-fifth of the planet's fresh water—is endangered through the clearing of rain forests, stripping of entire ecosystems for mines, and damming of rivers. Among the people of Brazil there is extensive poverty and inequality, exacerbated by the country's weak and uneven economic situation. Moreover, the geography, climate, economy, and poverty combine to place large segments of the population at risk for a wide range of viral, bacterial, and fungal infections and diseases—typhus, yellow fever, tuberculosis, hepatitis, intestinal worms, dengue, Chagas' disease, filariasis, and schistosomiasis to name but a few.

What few people outside of Brazil realize, furthermore, and what even most Brazilians are unaware of, is the extent to which HIV and AIDS are a problem in this great South American nation. In fact, at the closing of the millennium and moving into the twenty-first century, Brazil ranked second only to the United States in the number of reported cases of AIDS. As in the U.S., AIDS in Brazil was initially believed to be a disease of middle-class gay men. But as the epidemic expanded and the number of cases among women, heterosexual men, injection drug users, and children increased, efforts were mobilized by the country's Ministry of Health to curtail the spread of the disease. But because of Brazil's extensive poverty and inequality, its fragile economic situation, and limited network of health services, the scarce prevention/intervention resources targeted only the most visible at risk populations—gay men, sailors, prostitutes, and street children. Virtually forgotten were Brazil's hidden drug users, as well as the tens of millions of individuals living in the country's thousands of *favelas* or shantytowns, which are a characteristic part of almost every Brazilian city. Also forgotten were the scores of indigent residents of the *asfalto*, the "asphalt city," the low-income/high-crime areas of urban centers beyond the slopes of the *favelas*.

Within the context of these opening remarks *Sex, Drugs, and HIV/AIDS in Brazil* examines the emergence of AIDS as a global epidemic and, particularly in Brazil, its linkages to drug use and the sexual culture, and its epidemiology in such populations as cocaine users, "street children," and male transvestite prostitutes. Special attention, furthermore, is focused on an HIV/AIDS community outreach program established in Rio de Janeiro, which represented the first such prevention/intervention effort in all of Brazil targeting indigent cocaine users. This six-year initiative was funded by the Community Research Branch of the U.S. National Institute on Drug Abuse, and carried out by the authors of this book through collaborative arrangements between the State University of Rio de Janeiro, the University of Miami School of Medicine, and the University of Delaware.

James A. Inciardi
Hilary L. Surratt
Paulo R. Telles

Acknowledgments

The total number of debts that are incurred during a project of this scope is surprisingly large. In this regard, our first acknowledgment must go to our colleagues and staff who participated in this project, particularly those at the Center for Drug and Alcohol Studies at the University of Delaware, the Comprehensive Drug Research Center at the University of Miami School of Medicine, and the Núcleo de Estudos e Pesquisas em Atenção ao Uso de Drogas of the State University of Rio de Janeiro. Second, acknowledgment must also be given to the staff at the Community Research Branch of the National Institute on Drug Abuse who were responsible for the funding and monitoring of the research. Third, and most importantly, we wish to thank the many hundreds of clients from the *favelas* and *asfalto* in Rio de Janeiro without whom this project never would have succeeded.

J.A.I.
H.L.S.
P.R.T.

1

HIV, AIDS, and Drug Use

When the noted French poet and chronicler Jean Froissart wrote at the close of the 14th century that "a third of the world has died," he was reflecting on the how the Black Death had ravaged the population of Europe, and how little medieval medicine had to offer in its fight against epidemic diseases. Now, at the beginning of the 21st century, modern medical science is attempting to register progress against AIDS—the most dramatic, pervasive, and tragic epidemic of our time.

Given the media attention to AIDS, and to HIV—the virus that causes AIDS—it is likely that major segments of the world's population have at least heard of the disease. However, other than the basic ways that AIDS is transmitted, the majority of people in most communities are unfamiliar with the specifics of the disease continuum.

HIV, or *human immunodeficiency virus*, is a "retrovirus," a type of infectious agent that had previously been identified as causing many animal diseases. HIV destroys the body's immune system, and is transmitted when virus particles or infected cells gain direct access to the bloodstream. This can occur through all forms of sexual intercourse, using contaminated hypodermic needles and injection equipment, contact with contaminated blood and blood products, and the passing of the virus from infected mothers to their unborn or newborn children. Within this context, HIV causes a continuum of conditions associated with immune dysfunction, and AIDS, or acquired immune deficiency syndrome, is best described as a severe manifestation of infection with HIV.

Given the mechanisms of infection, the population groups having the highest rates of HIV and AIDS include men who have sex with other men, persons who share injection equipment, and recipients of blood products. In the United States, Brazil, and the majority of other Western nations, men who have sex with men and injection drug users represent the vast bulk of known AIDS cases, with other members of the AIDS caseload reflecting relatively small numbers. However, the heterosexual spread of HIV is increasing, particularly in those locales where rates of injection drug use are high. Elsewhere in the world, especially in many developing nations, heterosexual spread is the major route of transmission.

The Emergence of the Epidemic

AIDS was first described as a new and distinct clinical entity during the late spring and early summer of 1981 (CDC 1981a, 1981b; Gottlieb et al. 1981; Masur et al. 1981). First, clinical investigators in Los Angeles reported five cases to the U.S. Centers for Disease Control of *Pneumocystis carinii* pneumonia (PCP) among gay men. None of these patients had an underlying disease that might have been associated with PCP or a history of treatment for a compromised immune system. All, however, had other clinical manifestations and laboratory evidence of immunosuppression. Second, and within a month, 26 cases of Kaposi's sarcoma (KS) were reported among homosexual men in New York and California.

What was so unusual was that prior to these reports, the appearance of both PCP and KS in populations of previously healthy young men was unprecedented. PCP is an infection caused by the parasite *P. carinii*, heretofore seen almost exclusively in cancer and transplant patients receiving immunosuppressive drugs. Prior to the age of AIDS, *Pneumocystis carinii* pneumonia was one of the perhaps thousands of malevolent microorganisms that always lurked on the fringes of human existence. PCP was first observed in guinea pigs and identified in 1909 and 1910 by Brazilian virologists. In 1956, it was diagnosed for the first time among immunosuppressed patients (Hughes 1979; Golden 1989).

Kaposi's sarcoma, a cancer or tumor of the blood vessel walls and typically appearing as blue-violet to brownish skin blotches, had been quite rare in the United States—occurring primarily in elderly men, usually of Mediterranean or Jewish origin. Like PCP, furthermore, KS had also been reported among organ transplant recipients and others receiving immunosuppressive therapy. "Sarcoma" is a medical term describing a tumor that is often malignant, and Kaposi's sarcoma has been observed in a number of non-AIDS populations. First described in 1872 by the Viennese dermatologist Moritz Kaposi as a "multiple pigmented sarcoma of the skin," it was an extremely rare malignancy for over a century in both the United States and Europe. Clinically, it appeared most frequently as a tumor of the feet and lower extremities. It was not accompanied by immune suppression, other than the expected immunological attrition associated with aging.

The fact that both PCP and KS had been reported among patients receiving immunosuppressive therapy quickly led to the hypothesis that the increased occurrences of the two disorders in gay men were due to some underlying immune system dysfunction. This hypothesis was further supported by the incidence among gays of "opportunistic infections"—infections caused by microorganisms that rarely generate disease in persons with normal immune defense mechanisms. The occurrence of Kaposi's sarcoma, *P. carinii*, and/or other opportunistic infections in a person with unexplained immune dysfunction is why the affliction became known as the "acquired immune deficiency syndrome," or more simply, AIDS.

With the recognition that the vast majority of the early cases of this new clinical syndrome involved gay men, it seemed logical that the causes might be related to the lifestyle unique to that population. The so-called sexual revolution of the 1960s and 1970s was accompanied not only by greater carnal permissiveness among both heterosexuals and gays, but also by a more positive social acceptance of homosexuality in many communities. The emergence of commercial bathhouses and other outlets for sexual contacts among gays further increased promiscuity, with self-selected segments of the male gay population viewing promiscuity as a facet of "gay liberation." In fact, among many early patients diagnosed with AIDS, much of their sexual recreation with multiple partners typically occurred within the anonymity of the bathhouses with similarly promiscuous men. Some had had as many as 20,000 sexual contacts and more than 1,100 sex partners. And to complicate matters, active gay men with multiple sex partners were manifesting high rates of sexually transmitted diseases—gonorrhea, syphilis, genital herpes, anal warts, and hepatitis B (Rompalo and Handsfield 1989).

Because of this, it is not surprising that such factors as frequent exposure to semen, rectal exposure to semen, the body's exposure to amyl nitrite and butyl nitrite (better known as "poppers," and used to enhance sexual pleasure and performance), and/or a high frequency of sexually transmitted diseases were themselves considered potential causes of AIDS.

Yet while it was apparent that AIDS was a new disease, most of the gay lifestyle factors were not particularly new, having changed only in a relative sense. As such, it was difficult to immediately single out specific behaviors that might be related to the emerging epidemic. Nevertheless, in the minds of much of America AIDS was an immunity disease linked to homosexual practices and the homosexual condition. However, within a brief period of time, the notion that AIDS was some form of "gay plague" was quickly extinguished, at least within the public health community. The disease was suddenly being reported in other populations, such as intravenous and other injection drug users, blood transfusion patients, and hemophiliacs (CDC 1982). What these reports suggested to the scientific community was that an infectious etiology for AIDS had to be considered.

When AIDS cases began to emerge in other populations—among individuals who had been injected with blood or blood products, but had no other expected risk factors—the transmission vectors for the disease became somewhat clearer. Such cases were confirmed first among people with hemophilia, followed by blood transfusion recipients, and injection drug users who shared hypodermic needles. Then, when there were documented cases of AIDS among the heterosexual partners of male injection drug users, it became increasingly evident that AIDS was a sexually transmitted disease, and that "sexual preference" was not the element that placed people at risk (Giudici-Fettner 1987).

In 1983 and 1984, scientists at the Institute Pasteur in Paris and the National Institutes of Health in the United States identified and isolated the cause of AIDS—human T-Cell lymphotropic virus, Type III (HTLV-III), as it was called in the United States, or lymphadenophy-associated virus (LAV), as it was known by French scientists. Later, this virus was renamed "human immunodeficiency virus," more commonly known as HIV.

Subsequent to the discovery of HIV, an early priority was to fully verify its association with the diseases in question. Using a variety of different laboratory tests, researchers in virology and molecular biology searched for antibodies against HIV in the blood of AIDS patients. Ultimately, they found that almost 100 percent of AIDS patients had HIV antibodies (Institute of Medicine 1986). The presence of specific antibodies in the blood indicates that a previous infection registered on the body's immune system. The antibody molecules that remain in the bloodstream act as scouts, so to speak: if the virus appears again, the scouts recognize it immediately and attempt to prevent it from getting a foothold.

This research led, in 1985, to the widespread availability of a commercial test for antibodies to HIV. The basic test is an enzyme-linked immunosorbent assay (ELISA). More commonly known as ELISA, it is *not* a test for AIDS, nor does it even detect the presence of the virus itself. What the test does indicate is whether HIV has been noticed by an individual's immune system.

Modes of HIV Transmission

HIV has been isolated from blood, semen, saliva, urine, tears, breast milk, vaginal secretions, lung fluid, and cerebrospinal fluid (McCoy and Inciardi 1995). Because HIV has been identified in these fluids does not, however, mean that they are all important to transmission. Laboratory findings, along with overwhelming empirical observations, support the scientific conclusion that the major routes of HIV transmission are through human blood and sexual activities involving the exchange of semen and vaginal fluids.

Transmission among Men Who Have Sex with Men

Among men who have sex with other men, HIV infection can be transmitted in two basic ways—sexually and through direct contact with infected blood. Gay and bisexual men generally acquire HIV infection through sexual contact, and the risk of acquisition of infection depends on two variables: (1) the probability of exposure to an infected partner and (2) the probability of transmission from the infected partner (McCoy and Inciardi 1995).

The first variable, that sexual contact with a person known to be infected with HIV is associated with transmission, has been well documented (Polk et al. 1987). There is ample epidemiologic evidence that during homosexual intercourse, the virus is transmitted from the penis of the insertive partner into the anus and rectum of the receptive partner. The second variable, the risk of effective transfer of the virus, is not quite as easy to assess, for it depends on the specific sexual practices and whether the virus in the body fluid of the infected donor comes into contact with an available receptor cell in the recipient. What is clear, however, is that almost all sexual acts may transmit the virus. In some of the major HIV prevalence studies, unprotected receptive anal intercourse has been the major mode of transmission when other risk factors, including numbers of sex partners, were controlled for (Winkelstein et al. 1989). Similarly, unprotected receptive anal intercourse has been shown to be the primary mode of transmission of HIV in all cohort studies in which seroconversion (the initial development of antibodies after contact with HIV) has been analyzed during follow-up (Winkelstein et al. 1989). There is the potential for HIV to be transmitted during oral-genital sex, but the risk is considerably less than through anal sex (Edwards and Carne 1998).

In addition to receptive anal intercourse, there are two other modes of HIV transmission among gay men, both involving the direct transfer of infected blood. The first is associated with blood transfusion, but few of these cases have been reported. The second involves the sharing of infected drug paraphernalia among gay men who are also injection drug users.

Going one step further, there is the matter of "cofactors." These include any physical conditions, behavioral practices, or microbiological agents that facilitate the transmission of HIV. Two major categories of cofactors have been investigated: (1) those that might affect acquisition of HIV before or during sexual contact (such as foreplay and other ancillary sexual practices) and (2) those of a more general nature having the potential to enhance susceptibility.

There are two types of ancillary sexual practices among men who have sex with men of interest here:

1.   those that are likely to disrupt the sensitive tissues in the rectum, thereby facilitating infection; and
2.   those interfering with judgment that might render sex partners less likely to take precautions against acquiring infection.

The anus is a sensitive area, which, apart from its proximity to the genitals, appears to be intimately involved in both eliciting and responding to sexual stimuli. Some people react to anal stimulation erotically; others are indifferent to it, or find it repugnant. It is not an exclusively gay and bisexual male practice, for it occurs in heterosexual relations as well. In fact, in some cultures it is quite common as an alternative to vaginal intercourse (Parker 1991). In either case, the tissues inside the rectum are highly delicate, and minor tearing of these sensitive membranes is possible during any form of anal intercourse. Even when lubricants are used, extremely vigorous intercourse can cause rectal trauma. Moreover, not uncommon during sexual activity is the insertion of fingers and dildos into the rectum, and again, the potential for trauma exists.

An even greater likelihood for rectal injury exists with "fisting"—anal penetration by the fist, and sometimes by the forearm as well, through the rectum and possibly into the sigmoid colon (Browning 1993:84). A sharp fingernail can leave a deep cut in the rectum that can take weeks to heal. A fist ramming into the sigmoid colon—a part of the intestine several inches up from the anus—is even more problematic. The tissue lining the sigmoid colon has the consistency and delicacy of wet paper towels. In some people the area can expand to accommodate a fist, bleeding can result, and infection is likely.

Practices that interfere with judgment, which might render sex partners less likely to take precautions against acquiring infection, revolve around the use of psychoactive drugs. The three drugs of most significance are the nitrite inhalants, alcohol, and cocaine.

The nitrites—principally amyl and butyl nitrite—are liquid compounds that were first introduced into medicine more than a century ago for the treatment of angina (heart pain). They have had other therapeutic uses, as muscle relaxants and vasodilators (for increasing blood flow through capillaries). The primary effect of these drugs is the relaxation of all smooth muscles in the body, including those in the blood vessels, thus allowing a greater flow of oxygenated blood to the brain

(Nickerson 1975). Amyl and butyl nitrite were originally supplied in glass vials (ampules), which were broken open (or popped or snapped open) and inhaled, and hence, acquired such street names in the United States as "poppers" and "snappers." They are quick-acting drugs, taking effect in 15 to 30 seconds, with a duration of two to three minutes. On inhalation, there is a distinct "rush" (the initial flood of pleasure, with quickened heart rate, felt soon after the ingestion of certain psychoactive drugs).

The recreational popularity of the nitrites results from their reputation as aphrodisiacs. To gain this effect, they are usually inhaled just prior to orgasm. According to some observers, however, the reported intensification and prolongation of orgasm may be an illusion. The rush, involving dizziness and giddiness, may cause a reduction of social and sexual inhibitions along with time distortion. Clearly, this combination may lead to a sense of prolonged orgasm (Louria 1970; Seymour and Smith 1987:40). On the other hand, an increased flow of blood to the genitals may indeed increase sensitivity to sexual activity.

For years, the nitrites were sold over-the-counter, but reports of widespread abuse in the U.S. during the 1960s resulted in their reclassification as prescription drugs. Since that time, however, other volatile nitrites containing isomers of the nitrites have become available as sexual enhancers.

Alcohol's relationship to high-risk sexual behavior has been well documented. In several studies of gay men, for example, alcohol use combined with sexual activity was found to be strongly associated with such risky practices as receptive anal intercourse, multiple anonymous sex partners, and lack of condom use (Gordis 1992). Similarly, cocaine has long since had a reputation for being a spectacular aphrodisiac: it is believed to create sexual desire, to heighten it, to increase sexual endurance, and to cure frigidity and impotence (Inciardi 1992:93–94).

There is a rather wide range of concurrent or prior infections that represent cofactors of a more general nature that have the potential to enhance susceptibility to HIV. Of most significance are infections associated with enteric and sexually transmitted diseases. Syphilis, gonorrhea, and anal and genital warts and herpes have been associated with HIV infection. Then there are the enteric diseases—particularly amebiasis, giardiasis, and shigella—which are caused by organisms that lodge themselves in the intestinal tract. Such infections tend to be common in the gay community, typically the result of anal intercourse, which puts an individual in contact with his partner's fecal matter. An even more direct mechanism of ingesting the parasitic spoor associated with these conditions is through the practice of "rimming" (oral-anal intercourse)—the act of placing one's tongue into the anus of another (Silverstein and Picano

1992:156–157). The resulting parasitic infections often cause chronic diar-rhea, which can bring on significant immune suppression. These para-sitic infections pose yet another immunosuppressive risk for gay men, for many antiparasitic drugs can have adverse effects on the immune sys-tem. Decreased immune response, furthermore, increases one's suscepti-bility to HIV infection.

Transmission among Injection Drug Users

The sharing of hypodermic needles, syringes, and other injection equip-ment is the most likely route of HIV transmission among injection drug users. The vector is the exchange of the blood of the previous user that is lodged in the needle, the syringe, or some other part of the "works" (drug paraphernalia). Levels of risk vary, however, depending on the particular injection practice. Of lesser risk, for example, is "skin-popping"—the intradermal (into the skin), subcutaneous (under the skin), or intramuscular (into the muscle) injection of cocaine, narcotics, and other drugs. Skin-popping (or simply popping) is a common method of heroin use by experimenters and "tasters" (novice and casual users) who mistakenly believe that addiction cannot occur through this route (Kaplan 1983:10; Baden 1975).

At the opposite end of the risk spectrum is "booting," a process involv-ing the use of a syringe to draw blood from the user's arm, the mixing of the drawn blood with the drug already taken into the syringe, and the in-jection of the blood/drug mixture into the vein. Many injection drug users believe that this practice potentiates a drug's effects. Importantly, however, booting leaves traces of blood in the needle and syringe, thus placing subsequent users of the injection equipment at risk (Inciardi 1990). Although most injection drug users are generally aware of the risks associated with booting and needle sharing, they are often ignored. Moreover, little thought is typically given to the risks associated with other aspects of the injection process.

Virological studies have indicated that HIV can survive in ordinary tap water for extended periods of time. In a series of experiments conducted at the Laboratory of Tumor Cell Biology, National Institutes of Health, for example, infectious cell-free virus could be recovered from dried material after up to three days at room temperature, and in an aqueous medium, virus survived longer than 15 days at room temperature (Resnick et al. 1986). Similar results were found in complementary studies conducted at the Institute Pasteur in Paris (Martin et al. 1985). Along comparable lines, researchers at the University of Miami School of Medicine demonstrated the viability of HIV in blood and cell culture medium in needles and sy-ringes at room temperatures up to 24 hours (Shapshak et al. 1994). The implication of these findings is that shared water used in the injection process represents a potential disease reservoir.

Injection drug users require water to both rinse their syringes and mix with their drugs to liquify them for injection. Rinsing, for example, is not necessarily for hygienic purposes, but to make sure a syringe does not become clogged with blood and drug residue, so that it can be used again. This rinse water is often shared, and as such, water contaminated through the rinsing of a syringe is used for rinsing other syringes and for mixing the drug. Similarly, "spoons," "cookers," and "cottons" are parts of the injection kit that also represent potential reservoirs of disease. Spoons and cookers are the bottle caps, spoons, baby food jars, and other small containers used for mixing the drug, while cottons refer to any materials placed in the spoon to filter out undissolved drug particles. Filtering is considered necessary since undissolved particles tend to clog injection equipment. The risks of HIV infection from spoons and cottons are due to their frequent sharing, even by drug users who carry their own syringes.

Viral contamination might also result from "front-loading" and "back-loading," techniques for distributing a drug solution among a drug injecting group (Grund et al. 1990). When front-loading, the drug is transferred from the syringe used for measuring by removing the needle from the receiving syringe and squirting the solution directly into its hub. Common in many urban "shooting galleries" (places where drugs are used and/or shared) is the intercontamination of drug doses through the mixing and front-loading of "speedball" (heroin and cocaine). Since heroin is "cooked" (heated in an aqueous solution), whereas cocaine is not during its preparation for injecting, separate containers are used for the mixing process. Those who share speedball draw the heroin into one syringe and the cocaine into another, remove the needle from the cocaine syringe and discharge the heroin into it through its hub, and return half the speedball mixture back into the syringe that originally contained the heroin. If either syringe contains virus at the start of such an operation, both are likely to contain it afterward (Inciardi and Page 1991).

The back-loading of speedball has also been observed in many shooting galleries. Back-loading involves essentially the same process, but the plunger, rather than the needle, is removed from the receiving syringe. Front-loading seems to be the preferred mixing/sharing method, with back-loading as a substitute when syringes with detachable needles are unavailable.

An alternative method of drug sharing is referred to by some drug injectors as "shooting back" and "drawing up." This practice has been observed in instances when every member of the drug sharing group has a syringe. After the heroin, cocaine, or speedball is thoroughly mixed, it is discharged from the mixing syringe into a common spoon, cap, or container. Each member of the sharing group then draws a specific amount.

For many decades, the sharing of injection equipment has been a prominent aspect of the subculture of the street drug scene in many parts of the world, and all of its associated practices are generally learned during initiation to drug use. A user's first episode of sharing is typically unplanned. Since novice injectors rarely have their own injection kit or "works," they often borrow a more experienced user's equipment. After becoming a regular user, association with a shooting or "running" partner may begin and sharing both drugs and needles may serve as a convenience and a symbol of friendship and trust. Since a shooting partner is often a lover, a surrogate family member, or a replacement family, refusing to share injection equipment could be viewed as an indication of mistrust. For shooting partners who are also sex partners, injecting drugs as a pair may serve as an even deeper symbol of emotional bonding. In addition, the mixing of blood while injecting and the booting of each other's blood is not uncommon, symbolizing a brotherhood or sisterhood or bond between running partners. The risks of such ritual blood exchanges, of course, are obvious, and are likely responsible for HIV and scores of other infections.

Heterosexual Transmission

At present, the biological variables that determine HIV "infectivity" (the tendency to spread from host to host) and "susceptibility" (the tendency for a host to become infected) are incompletely understood. HIV has been isolated from the semen of infected men, and it appears that it may be harbored in the cells of pre-ejaculated fluids or sequestered in inflammatory lesions (Fischl et al. 1987). Furthermore, there is evidence that women can harbor HIV in vaginal and cervical secretions at varying times during the menstrual cycle (Vogt et al. 1987).

The evidence for sexual transmission of HIV among gay and bisexual men through anal intercourse, and to women through vaginal intercourse, has been well documented. However, although there is the potential for viral transmission from female secretions, the absolute amounts of virus in these secretions appear to be relatively low. The efficiency of transmission of male-to-female versus female-to-male is likely affected by the relative infectivity of these different secretions, as well as sex during menses, specific sexual practices, the relative integrity of skin and mucosal surfaces involved, and the presence of other sexually transmitted diseases. Given this, there are a number of issues to be examined when considering the heterosexual transmission of HIV from men to women and from women to men. Of particular interest are the biological variables, risk factors and cofactors, and particular sexual practices among those populations with the highest rates of heterosexual transmission.

Male-to-Female Transmission. Heterosexual contact per se is an essential but not a sufficient condition for the transmission of HIV. A variety of studies have demonstrated, for example, that an average of only 15 percent of the women who are steady partners of HIV-infected men acquire the infection, despite repeated sexual exposures (Johnson et al. 1988). Thus, the risk of contracting HIV through a single sexual exposure is not particularly high in the great majority of instances (Holmberg et al. 1989). However, there is evidence that although some people remain uninfected after hundreds of episodes of unprotected sex, others have become infected after only one or just a few sexual encounters (Padian et al. 1988). These observations would suggest that there are cofactors that affect the likelihood of HIV transmission.

Three groups of factors influencing the probability of acquiring HIV through male-to-female sexual contact have been suggested: (1) sexual behavior and risk duration (2) infectiousness of the HIV positive partner, and (3) host susceptibility (Johnson and Laga 1988). Looking first at sexual behavior and risk duration, it was noted earlier in this chapter that the potential for infection among gay men increases with the number of partners and the frequency of sexual intercourse. However, a majority of early studies of heterosexual transmission failed to show a relationship between risk of infection and either the frequency of sexual intercourse or the duration of a relationship with an infected partner (Peterman et al. 1988; Johnson et al. 1988; Laga et al. 1988; Goedert et al. 1988). These results were surprising and counterintuitive, and may have been the result of measurement error, improper statistical analysis, and the failure to account for other factors.

More recent investigations have found that the number of exposures to an infected partner is indeed associated with transmission. With regard to the infectiousness of the seropositive partner, a higher rate of infection among the female partners of men in advanced clinical stages of HIV disease has been well documented. This is likely due to the fact that the declining immune function allows the virus to replicate, unchecked, in an HIV positive individual, and as such, there are higher concentrations of HIV (termed "viral load") in such bodily fluids as blood and semen. Studies also document that although the transmission of HIV between male and female partners is not always certain with any given exposure, considerable risk is always present in either direction, and can increase dramatically depending on the type and frequency of the sexual contacts, and the immunological state of the partners (McCoy and Inciardi 1995:96–97).

Female-to-Male Transmission.   Female-to-male sexual transmission of HIV is supported by biological plausibility, equal numbers of male and female AIDS cases in some African countries, case reports of males with no risk factors other than heterosexual intercourse, and seroconversion of male sex partners of infected women that occurred while the couples were being studied prospectively. In terms of the biological plausibility of female-to-male transmission, it has been argued that since other sexually transmitted diseases are bidirectional in nature, it is not unreasonable to assume that HIV can spread in the same manner. A number of studies have documented that African and Indian men who have multiple female sex partners or sexual contact with prostitutes are at high risk for becoming infected with HIV (Bond et al. 1997). The most persuasive case reports of female-to-male transmission have been those in which (1) the female acquired the infection from a transfusion or organ transplant and her male partner (without other known risk factors) subsequently seroconverted, and (2) where a sequential chain of male-to-female-to-male transmission was observed.

Although significant numbers of female-to-male infections have been documented in Africa (Bond et al. 1997), such a mode of transmission has been reported only infrequently in other parts of the world. Several explanations have been offered for the differences in female-to-male transmission rates in Africa as compared to Europe and North and South American countries. A number of researchers have suggested that the infrequent documentation of heterosexual transmission from women to men in Europe and the Americas may be a function of the history of the epidemic. They suggest that because the initial phase was largely confined to gay men and injection drug users, the number of infected women was low during that time, and therefore the possibility of female-to-male transmission was small.

By contrast, there is considerable evidence of viral transmission by HIV-infected African prostitutes to their male customers (Bond et al. 1997). A number of factors contribute to this. Among African prostitutes and their customers there appear to be significant proportions with untreated STDs, including genital ulcers, and these appear to increase men's susceptibility to HIV. In addition, several studies have noted that sex workers in the West are more conscious of STDs and are more likely to use safer sexual practices (e.g., vaginal and anal sex with condoms) with customers than their counterparts in Africa.

What all of this suggests is that AIDS prevention and intervention efforts must be dynamic. In any given locale they must address specific community circumstances and contingencies, cultural differences, perceptions of vulnerability, and the social roles of those at risk.

The Global Epidemiology of HIV and AIDS

At the close of 1999, a total of just over 2.2 million AIDS cases had been officially reported to the World Health Organization since the beginning of the epidemic (WHO 1999). Nearly all countries have reporting systems in place, but these systems vary greatly in the proportion of AIDS cases that are reported. Most industrialized nations report all cases, while others report only a small proportion because of underdiagnosis, incomplete enumeration, reporting delays, or deliberate underreporting for public relations and/or political reasons.

As illustrated in Table 1.1, approximately half the reported AIDS cases came from the Americas. In fact, worldwide, the United States ranked first in the number of reported cases (n=717,430), followed by Brazil (n=163,355). Other countries with significant numbers of cases included Thailand, France, Spain, Italy, Mexico, and several African nations. The data in Table 1.1 also illustrate the lags in reporting—with several countries one or more years behind, and no reports from Somalia and the United Arab Emirates since the beginning of the 1990s.

In addition to AIDS, the World Health Organization (WHO) and the United Nations Program on HIV/AIDS (UNAIDS) estimated that at the end of 1998 some 33.4 million people were living with HIV or AIDS (see Figure 1.1), and that during 1998 alone some 5.8 million women and children were infected with HIV (see Figure 1.2). But as illustrated in these graphics and in the discussions below, the epidemic is spreading at a differential rate around the world.

HIV/AIDS in Africa

Of people living with HIV around the world, six in every ten adult men, eight in every ten adult women, and more than nine of every ten children infected are in sub-Saharan Africa. Of the global estimate of 16,000 new HIV infections each day, almost half occur in sub-Saharan Africa (UN-AIDS 1998). Such factors as growing economic disparity, social and cultural uprooting linked to intense migration, insufficiencies in prevention and care programs and power gaps linked to gender, age, and economic differences continue to fuel HIV epidemics across the continent (UN-AIDS 1998).

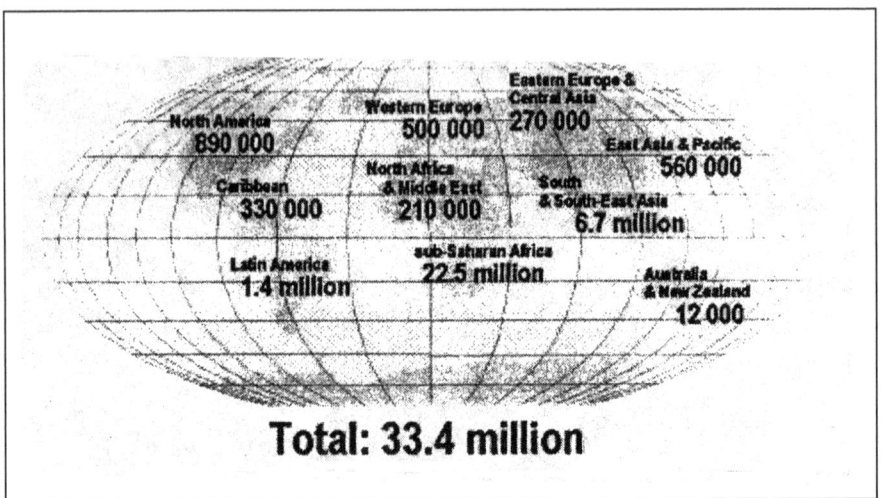

FIGURE 1.1   Adults and Children Living with HIV/AIDS (1998)

Africa is not uniformly affected by HIV/AIDS, however, for there appear to be a mosaic of epidemics progressing with varied intensity and velocity on various parts of the continent. For example, in prenatal clinics of several cities in southern Africa, up to 45 percent of women tested during pregnancy carry HIV, a rate ten or more times greater than in pregnant women seen at urban prenatal clinics in most countries in Central or West Africa.

Heterosexual contacts and mother-to-infant transmission of HIV account for the vast majority of HIV infections in the region. Anecdotal evidence supports the assertion that sex between men does occur in the region, particularly in single-sex male communities around industrial sites and in prisons. However, documented evidence of such a pattern of sexual behavior is lacking. The rising availability of injectable drugs such as heroin, especially at new transit points for drug trafficking, creates an additional risk for the spread of HIV in sub-Saharan Africa. The transmission of HIV infection through unscreened blood transfusions continues to be a concern in several countries in sub-Saharan Africa. In this region in 1995, over 2.5 million blood transfusions were administered—most of them to women and children—and of those, nearly a quarter had not been screened for HIV antibodies (UNAIDS 1998). Similarly, occupa-

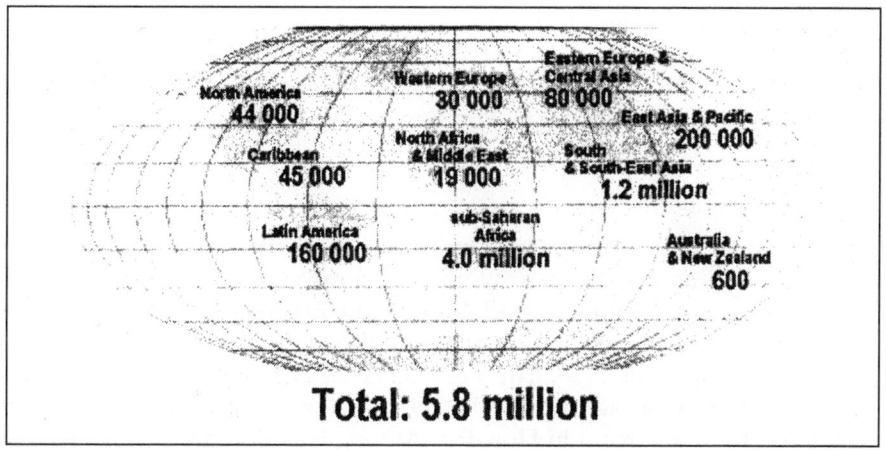

FIGURE 1.2   Adults and Children Newly Infected with HIV During 1998

tional exposure to HIV by health care workers has received only minimal attention.

HIV/AIDS in Asia/Pacific

With over 60 percent if the world's population, the Asia-Pacific region presents a wide diversity of HIV-related risk environments, in terms of behavioral, political, and cultural factors. Nevertheless, it is possible to classify the differing patterns of HIV transmission into broad categories, based on available surveillance data. In Australia and New Zealand, for example, the overwhelming majority of HIV infections has resulted from men having sex with men, although the incidence of transmission via this route has declined substantially in recent years. In a few countries, such as Thailand, Cambodia, and parts of Myanmar and India, heterosexual transmission has been extensive, mediated through large-scale sex industries but extending now to the regular partners of sex workers' male clients (UNAIDS 1998).

Some Asia-Pacific nations have HIV epidemics among injection drug users, with limited associated heterosexual transmission. These include Thailand, Malaysia, Vietnam, and some areas of India and China. Other nations have limited, but well-documented spread of HIV infections, such as the Philippines, Indonesia, Japan, and South Korea. Several countries have not reported substantial numbers of HIV infections, but do not appear to have comprehensive, ongoing surveillance systems, including Papua New Guinea, Pakistan, and Bangladesh.

HIV/AIDS in North America

Approximately 40,000 new HIV infections occur in the United States each year, more than one-third in women and more than two-thirds among ethnic minorities. An estimated 400,000 to 650,000 persons in the United States were living with HIV without AIDS-defining diseases or symptoms at the close of 1998. The prevalence of HIV infection in men who have sex with men attending STD clinics ranges from 3.7 percent in the Midwest to 31.4 percent in Houston. Among injection drug users, HIV infection is concentrated along the East Coast and in the South, with highs of 32.2 percent in Baltimore, 28.5 percent in New York City, and 25 percent in Atlanta. The geographic distribution of HIV infection in childbearing women mirrors that of injection drug users, with the highest rates along the Atlantic coast and in the South. Extreme differences exist in the distribution of HIV infection by race/ethnicity; prevalence is 22 times higher in blacks than whites in New York and 16 times higher in Florida.

Of the estimated 50,000 to 54,000 cumulative HIV infections that occurred in Canada since the beginning of the epidemic, 63.1 percent were among men who have sex with men, 4.2 percent among gay and bisexual injectors, 17.7 percent among injection drug users, 13.7 percent among heterosexuals, and 1.3 percent among recipients of blood or blood products. HIV prevalence among drug injectors has increased dramatically in many Canadian cities in recent years (in Ottawa, for example, from 10 percent in 1993 to 21 percent in 1997).

HIV/AIDS in Latin America and the Caribbean

The Latin American and Caribbean region encompasses the countries and territories in the Western Hemisphere from Mexico south and east to the tip of the Southern Cone of South America. The aggregate population of the 44 countries in the region totals some 476 million people, 8.4 percent of the global total of 5.7 billion people. An estimated 1.6 million people are living with HIV/AIDS in Latin America and the Caribbean, equivalent to 5.4 percent of the total number of people around the world living with HIV/AIDS (UNAIDS 1998).

HIV epidemics in Latin America and the Caribbean reflect the heterogeneity of HIV epidemics worldwide: they differ from country to country and within countries. In Mexico, for example, sex between men is the main transmission route in major cities, and drug-related transmission has begun in the northwestern part of the country; heterosexual transmission is more common along the southern border and in rural areas. Transfusion-related infections have diminished dramatically in the last eight years.

Five countries of Central America appear to have epidemics that are either in an early phase or show slow growth. In Honduras, however, the epidemic appears to be well established. Although Honduras accounts for only 17 percent of the subregion's population, it has reported more than half of the AIDS cases from Central America. Infections in this area are seen mainly in capitals and major cities, where commercial sex plays a role, while rural cases are related to migration. Since 1987 there has been a dramatic shift to heterosexual transmission and to younger population groups.

In Haiti and the Dominican Republic, HIV is spreading mostly through heterosexual intercourse (UNAIDS 1998). These countries have reported HIV prevalence rates among pregnant women attending prenatal clinics ranging from 1 to 9 percent while Cuba is showing rapidly increasing infection among men who have sex with men. In the other countries of the Caribbean, a few epidemics are evident among injection drug users as well as gay and bisexual men. Heterosexual transmission, however, has been the main route since 1986, and HIV prevalence in pregnant women ranges from 1 to 7 percent. Tourism and high population mobility characterize these island nations, and both factors can influence the spread of HIV.

The predominant mode of transmission in the five countries of the Andean area continues to be sexual contact among men who have sex with men. In general, HIV prevalence among pregnant women is less than 1 percent, although it has shown an increasing trend in the last few years. This slow increase probably reflects transmission from injection drug users to their female sex partners.

A mosaic of transmission routes accounts for the more than 500,000 HIV infections and 163,355 AIDS cases currently estimated in Brazil. Transmission through drug injectors and gay and bisexual men has dominated so far, but there is a growing epidemic fueled by heterosexual transmission. In urban areas, HIV prevalence in pregnant women ranges from 1 to 5 percent. Prevalence among female sex workers is around 5 percent and among injection drug users from 15 to 60 percent. Overall, the epidemic is moving into younger, and more impoverished populations, and into the smaller cities in the interior of the country.

The Southern Cone of South America shows a mixed picture, but transmission occurs mainly among men who have sex with men and injection drug users. The epidemics are occurring in major urban areas. Argentina reports HIV prevalence now ranging from 1 to 3 percent among pregnant women and 6 to 11 percent among female sex workers (UNAIDS 1998). Uruguay also shows an epidemic concentrated on gay and bisexual men and injection drug users with some limited spread to the general population, while Chile and Paraguay show low-grade epidemics.

Overall, HIV in Latin America and the Caribbean is concentrated in populations living on the social and economic margins of society. HIV/AIDS has taken its greatest toll on men who have sex with men and injection drug users, and in some places there is clear evidence of increasing spread among the impoverished segments of society. Rising rates in women show that heterosexual transmission is becoming more prominent.

Postscript

The spread of HIV/AIDS has been cast as both an "epidemic" (occurring in a specific geographical area) and a "pandemic" (an epidemic occurring in many parts of the world at the same time). Similarly, the rapid infusion of drug use into modern, industrialized societies has also been referred to as an epidemic. The intersecting epidemics of both AIDS and injection drug use share something of a common history since the early 1980s as epidemiological research discerned the link between contaminated injection equipment and the acquisition of HIV infection. Thus, large, highly marginalized populations have been put at risk for HIV infection through the use of shared drug paraphernalia. At the same time, although prostitution has long since been a common source of income for scores of drug-dependent women, exchanges of sex for drugs, or for money to buy drugs, has become far more frequent among non–injection drug users. This has resulted in higher rates of HIV infection through heterosexual transmission among heroin and cocaine snorters and smokers. Drug injectors, snorters, and smokers appear in reasonably large numbers in urban settings throughout the industrialized world, especially in the United States and Brazil. In the chapters that follow, the epidemics of HIV and AIDS in Brazil are examined more closely, with a special focus on intervention initiatives targeting marginalized, indigent, drug-using populations.

TABLE 1.1   Global AIDS Cases

Country/Area	Number of Cases	Date of Report
Africa		
Algeria	410	15.11.99
Angola	2,433	26.03.99
Benin	2,813	06.06.98
Botswana	10,142	10.06.99
Burkina Faso	13,518	11.06.99
Burundi	12,014	30.06.99
Cameroon	18,986	29.10.99
Cape Verde	269	29.01.99
Central African Republic	7,016	30.05.97
Chad	10,121	03.06.99
Comoros	20	12.10.99
Congo	10,223	06.09.96
Côte d'Ivoire	49,532	30.08.99
Democratic Republic of the Congo	47,557	20.10.99
Djibouti	1,783	06.04.99
Egypt	215	04.08.99
Equatorial Guinea	321	03.11.98
Eritrea	6,873	30.06.99
Ethiopia	37,874	04.07.99
Gabon	1,660	31.12.97
Gambia	637	15.06.99
Ghana	29,546	20.05.99
Guinea	5,307	14.06.99
Guinea-Bissau	823	31.10.96
Kenya	81,492	28.09.98
Lesotho	7,317	31.12.98
Liberia	272	26.10.98
Libyan Arab Jamahiriya	32	25.05.99
Madagascar	37	07.10.99
Malawi	50,975	21.05.98
Mali	5,263	14.10.99
Mauritania	532	31.05.97
Mauritius	50	12.11.99
Morocco	510	30.06.98
Mozambique	10,863	25.03.99
Namibia	6,784	31.03.97
Niger	3,644	11.06.99
Nigeria	26,276	13.09.99
Réunion	166	31.12.95
Rwanda	15,903	31.12.97
São Tomé and Principe	70	14.10.99

(continues)

(continued)

TABLE 1.1   Global AIDS Cases

Country/Area	Number of Cases	Date of Report
Senegal	2,688	30.09.99
Seychelles	32	09.06.99
Sierra Leone	317	21.08.98
Somalia	13	31.12.90
South Africa	12,825	30.10.96
Sudan	2,735	05.10.99
Swaziland	3,528	15.07.99
Togo	10,827	08.03.99
Tunisia	519	21.07.99
Uganda	54,712	31.03.99
United Republic of Tanzania	112,052	11.08.99
Zambia	44,942	21.07.97
Zimbabwe	74,782	30.11.98
TOTAL	**800,251**	
Americas		
Anguilla	5	30.12.95
Antigua and Barbuda	96	31.05.99
Argentina	15,166	01.10.99
Bahamas	3,098	29.02.99
Barbados	1,043	16.09.99
Belize	198	30.04.97
Bermuda	346	15.11.99
Bolivia	179	16.04.97
Brazil	163,355	30.05.99
British Virgin Islands	16	31.10.98
Canada	15,935	31.08.98
Cayman Islands	24	31.05.99
Chile	2,821	31.03.99
Colombia	8,433	31.12.97
Costa Rica	1,580	15.11.99
Cuba	846	31.08.99
Dominica	87	15.11.99
Dominican Republic	4,733	10.09.99
Ecuador	872	28.02.98
El Salvador	2,378	15.11.99
French Guiana	641	31.12.97
Grenada	103	30.11.97
Guadeloupe	790	31.12.97
Guatemala	3,392	31.08.99
Guyana	1,053	31.10.98

TABLE 1.1   Global AIDS Cases

Country/Area	Number of Cases	Date of Report
Haiti	8,899	28.02.99
Honduras	8,217	28.01.98
Jamaica	2,975	15.11.99
Martinique	436	31.12.97
Mexico	39,675	31.05.99
Montserrat	8	31.05.99
Netherlands Antilles and Aruba	257	31.03.96
Nicaragua	182	15.11.99
Panama	1,942	15.11.99
Paraguay	424	15.07.98
Peru	8,940	30.09.99
Saint Kitts and Nevis	58	08.09.97
Saint Lucia	111	28.02.99
Saint Vincent and the Grenadines	139	28.02.99
Suriname	211	31.12.96
Trinidad and Tobago	2,613	02.07.97
Turks and Caicos Islands	39	03.11.93
USA	733,374	31.12.99
Uruguay	1,193	22.09.99
Venezuela	7,282	24.04.98
TOTAL	**1,044,165**	

Asia

Afghanistan	—	17.10.99
Armenia	15	02.11.99
Azerbaijan	12	02.11.99
Bahrain	70	28.06.99
Bangladesh	10	31.03.98
Bhutan	—	30.11.96
Brunei Darussalam	12	31.08.99
Cambodia	4,834	30.06.99
China	419	15.10.99
Cyprus	97	09.08.99
Democratic People's Republic of Korea	—	30.11.96
Georgia	27	02.11.99
Hong Kong Special Administrative Region of China	409	30.06.99
India	8,438	31.08.99

(continues)

(continued)

TABLE 1.1   Global AIDS Cases

Country/Area	Number of Cases	Date of Report
Indonesia	265	15.11.99
Iran	215	25.01.99
Iraq	108	18.04.99
Israel	548	02.11.99
Japan	2,066	27.06.99
Jordan	71	10.08.99
Kazakhstan	25	02.11.99
Kuwait	46	18.05.99
Kyrgyzstan	27	30.06.98
Lao People's Democratic Republic	105	07.10.99
Lebanon	147	02.03.99
Macao	17	30.06.99
Malaysia	2,894	30.06.99
Maldives	5	30.04.97
Mongolia	1	04.08.99
Myanmar	2,568	31.03.98
Nepal	261	30.06.99
Oman	367	11.08.99
Pakistan	173	24.05.99
Philippines	404	11.10.99
Qatar	93	10.06.99
Republic of Korea	147	10.10.99
Saudi Arabia	414	01.08.99
Singapore	545	15.10.99
Sri Lanka	93	11.02.99
Syrian Arab Republic	65	28.07.99
Tajiikistan	—	30.06.98
Thailand	128,606	31.10.99
Turkey	304	02.11.99
Turkmenistan	1	30.11.95
United Arab Emirates	8	28.02.91
Uzbekistan	7	02.11.99
Vietnam	2,736	07.08.99
West Bank and Gaza Strip	33	21.08.99
Yemen	156	25.02.99
TOTAL	**157,864**	
Europe		
Albania	11	02.11.99
Austria	1,915	02.11.99
Belarus	23	02.11.99

TABLE 1.1   Global AIDS Cases

Country/Area	Number of Cases	Date of Report
Belgium	2,599	02.11.99
Bosnia and Herzegovina	17	25.06.97
Bulgaria	60	02.11.99
Croatia	144	02.11.99
Czech Republic	125	02.11.99
Denmark	2,216	02.11.99
Estonia	22	02.11.99
Finland	294	02.11.99
France	49,421	02.11.99
Germany	18,239	02.11.99
Greece	1,964	02.11.99
Hungary	328	02.11.99
Iceland	50	02.11.99
Ireland	674	02.11.99
Italy	44,516	02.11.99
Latvia	37	02.11.99
Lithuania	26	02.11.99
Luxembourg	139	02.11.99
Malta	47	02.11.99
Monaco	40	30.11.99
Netherlands	5,054	02.11.99
Norway	638	02.11.99
Poland	794	02.11.99
Portugal	6,020	02.11.99
Republic of Moldova	23	02.11.99
Romania	5,928	02.11.99
Russian Federation	395	02.11.99
San Marino	14	02.11.99
Slovakia	22	02.11.99
Slovenia	81	02.11.99
Spain	54,964	02.11.99
Sweden	1,663	02.11.99
Switzerland	6,641	02.11.99
The Former Yugoslav Republic of Macedonia	29	02.11.99
Ukraine	1,022	02.11.99
United Kingdom	16,437	02.11.99
Yugoslavia, Federal Republic	806	02.11.99
TOTAL	**223,438**	

Oceania

| American Samoa | — | 27.09.98 |

(continues)

(continued)

TABLE 1.1   Global AIDS Cases

Country/Area	Number of Cases	Date of Report
Australia	8,140	30.06.99
Cook Islands	—	28.09.98
Fiji	8	11.08.98
French Polynesia	54	02.09.98
Guam	60	31.07.99
Kiribati	7	31.07.99
Mariana Islands	8	15.04.98
Marshall Islands	2	27.02.98
Micronesia, Federated States of	2	01.04.98
Nauru	—	20.10.97
New Caledonia and Dependencies	67	12.07.99
New Zealand	681	30.06.99
Niue	—	08.09.98
Palau	1	28.02.98
Papua New Guinea	618	31.03.99
Samoa	6	28.09.98
Solomon Islands	—	03.08.97
Tokelau	—	02.09.97
Tonga	14	03.09.98
Tuvalu	—	08.10.97
Vanuatu	—	21.09.98
Wallis and Futuna Islands	1	17.08.98
TOTAL	**9,669**	
WORLD TOTAL	**2,235,387**	

SOURCES: World Health Organization (1999) "Global AIDS Surveillance," *Weekly Epidemiological Record*, 47 (26 November): 401–402; Brazilian Ministry of Health (1999) *Boletim Epidemiologico AIDS* 12 (2): March/May; Centers for Disease Control, *HIV/AIDS Surveillance Report*, 11 (2) December.

2

Brazil and the Spectrum of HIV/AIDS

Brazil is a land of great diversity. It is the rain forests of Amazonia and the factories of São Paulo; it is the turquoise beaches of Bahia and the swamps and wetlands of the Pantanal; and it is Carnaval in Rio de Janeiro and the *gaúchos* of Rio Grande do Sul. And Brazil is Copacabana and Corcovado, the samba and *capoeira*, and soccer, *feijoada*, Pelé, *cachaça*, and world beat. And this diversity extends to Brazil's people, politics, economic situation, and culture. Brazil's sexual ecology, as well, reflects many complexities and contradictions. And, too, the country's proximity to the coca-growing regions of South America and its position along major drug smuggling and trafficking corridors has resulted in the development of significant drug problems among its peoples. As such, history, geography, culture, and economics have combined to place Brazil at high risk for the epidemics of both HIV/AIDS and drug use.

The People and Politics of Brazil

Brazil encompasses more than three million square miles of territory within its borders, an area roughly equivalent in size to the continental United States. Brazil's estimated population of some 160 million people outranks that of all of its Latin American neighbors, and makes it the sixth most populous country in the world. Moreover, the Brazilian population reflects a rich ethnic heritage, dating prior to the discovery of the New World.

It is believed that there were already between three and five million indigenous peoples living in Brazil when the Portuguese navigator Pedro Alvares Cabral first landed on its shores on April 22, 1500 (Bethell 1987). These local populations were almost immediately forced into plantation labor by the Portuguese, and by the middle of the 16th century their numbers had begun to decline because of exposure to European diseases. At the same time, the importation of African slaves began to increase substantially. In fact, scholars estimate that some 3 million Africans were transported to work the Brazilian sugar and coffee plantations before the abolition of slavery in 1888 (Burns 1980). In addition, the modern period of European emigration to Brazil began in 1850, with vast numbers of Italians, Portuguese, Spaniards, and Germans settling in Brazil. By the close of the 20th century, Brazil's population was 53 percent white, 34 percent multiracial, and 11 percent Afro-Brazilian. Of the remaining 2 percent, most are Asian immigrants. Combined, all of these populations contributed much to Brazil's unique cultural heritage. Regretfully, however, Brazil's original indigenous people currently number less than three hundred thousand, with the majority isolated in the Amazonas territory.

The southeastern region of Brazil, where the cities of São Paulo and Rio de Janeiro are situated, is by far the most heavily populated section of the country. Metropolitan São Paulo, the largest city in Brazil, is home to 16.6 million inhabitants, while Rio de Janeiro has a population of approximately 6 million. Brazil's highly diversified economy, which includes major industries (automobiles, aircraft, petrochemicals, steel, computers), and financial and banking services, is heavily concentrated in these urban centers. Agriculture and livestock are also highly productive sectors of the Brazilian economy, and are distributed throughout much of the country.

Politically as well, Brazil reflects a diverse history of governmental structures—colonialist rule, constitutional monarchy, military dictatorship, and modern democratic authority (Freyre 1986). The country was initially ruled from Lisbon as a Portuguese colonial territory until 1808, when the royal family fled the Napoleonic invasion and moved the government to Rio de Janeiro. In 1821, King João VI returned to Portugal, but his son remained and declared Brazil's independence and installed himself as its first emperor, Dom Pedro I. His empire was abolished in 1889, however, when a federal republic was established through a takeover by the military. Until 1930, the government functioned as a constitutional democracy, when yet another military coup placed Getúlio Dornelles Vargas in power. Vargas was elected president under the constitution of 1934, inaugurating Brazil's second republic. The Vargas administration was followed by a series of democratically elected presidents from 1945 to 1961, but in 1964 a military coup installed General Humberto Castelo Branco as president. The Branco takeover differed from the prior coups in that the military remained in power, rather than returning the government to civilian control as in the past. Under Branco's successors, Marshall Artur da Costa e Silva and General Emílio Garrastazú Medici (from

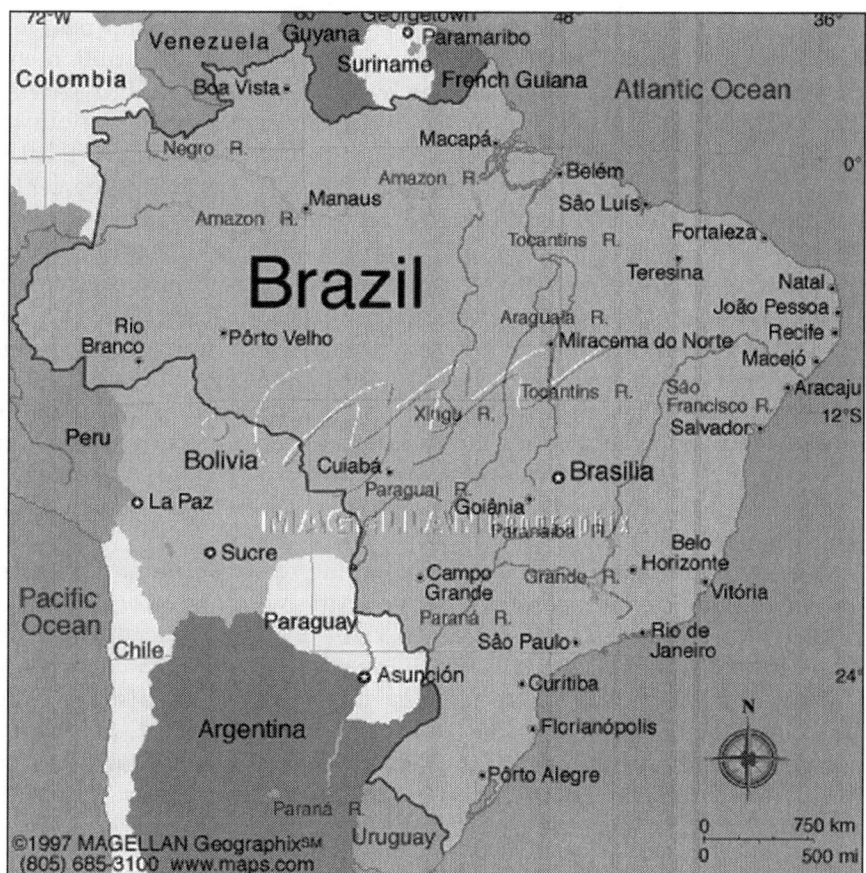

MAP 2.1   Brazil

1968 through 1973), Brazil experienced a period of severe repression marked by urban guerilla warfare, press censorship, arrests and kidnapping of opposition leaders, and widespread abuses by the military's secret police. When General Ernesto Geisel was named president in 1974, and in an attempt to stem rising opposition to military rule and remain in power, he established a process of liberalization or *abertura* that was continued by his successor, General João Baptista Figueiredo, which eventually culminated in the transition to a popularly elected government in 1989.

Economically, Brazil is often referred to as the land of perpetual promise, primarily because the country ranks near the bottom of the hemisphere in its standard of living, health status, and social indicators

(Willumsen and Giannetti da Fonseca 1997). Some 55 million people, a third of Brazil's total population, are under age 16, and 35 million children are living in families earning well under the minimum wage (UNICEF 1996). Almost half of all Brazilian families live below the poverty line (88% of the minimum wage), and almost a third are below the indigency line (53% of the minimum wage).[1] More than 18 percent of Brazil's population is illiterate, and 35 percent of children between ages 7 and 15 are not enrolled in school. In addition, with the exception of Haiti and Guatemala, malnutrition is more prevalent in Brazil than in any other Latin American or Caribbean nation (UNICEF 1996). According to official government statistics, 1,000 children die from hunger and malnutrition each day in Brazil. Moreover, Brazil's infant mortality rate in 1993 was 52 per 1,000 live births, one of the highest in Latin America and exceeded only by Peru (88) and Bolivia (98). In the poorest regions of the country and in impoverished areas near industrial centers, 10 percent of the children are expected to die before they reach five years of age (Martins 1993).

These discouraging numbers documenting the destitution of millions of Brazilians become even more bewildering when one considers that Brazil has a higher per capita GNP—$2,770—than any other Latin American country (except Uruguay). Brazil is a relatively wealthy country and possesses the tenth largest economy in the world, but the distribution of resources within its population is highly skewed. In fact, in 1996 the World Bank reported that for the second year in a row Brazil had the most lopsided income distribution in the world (*Latinamerica Press* 1996). For example, the wealthiest 20 percent of the population earned 65 percent of the country's total income, leaving only 12 percent for the poorest half. When Brazil is compared with other countries, the problem of inequity becomes even more obvious. The wealthiest 10 percent of the population earned 30 times more than the average income of the most impoverished 40 percent—a proportion that is ten-to-one in Argentina, nine to one in the United States, and only five to one in most European countries (*Latinamerica Press* 1996; Michaels 1993). Moreover, there is a staggering amount of land concentration in Brazil, with 43 percent of the total land area owned by 1 percent of the population (Raphael and Berkman 1992).

The striking economic disparity that exists between different segments of Brazilian society has its roots in regional inequalities and racial discrimination (Wood and Magno de Carvalho 1988). During Brazil's "Economic Miracle" of the 1970s, government funds and foreign loans flowed into the industries of the south, resulting in improved standards of living and employment opportunities in that area of the country. In the agricultural northern regions, however, the poverty rate increased 9 percent over this same time period (Raphael and Berkman 1992). Further, the aim of the Brazilian government to achieve "economic growth at all costs" led to a decrease in spending for health care, social programs, and educational initiatives. As a result, the proportion of malnourished children under age five increased from 13.7 percent in the late 1970s to 30.7 percent by the end of the 1980s.

With respect to economic disparity and racial inequality, Brazil is thought to have the largest black population of any country outside of Africa, with about 70 million people, or 46 percent of the total population being Afro-Brazilians (International Child Resource Institute 1994). Blacks in Brazil are typically overrepresented in the lowest income levels and represent the majority of the underemployed (International Child Resource Institute 1994). Several studies have documented that incomes of white Brazilians are, on average, twice that of black Brazilians (International Child Resource Institute 1994; Raphael and Berkman 1992; Wood and Magno de Carvalho 1988). In addition, a World Bank study found that almost 30 percent of Afro-Brazilian children live in households with incomes at the lowest wage levels (Tilak 1989).

An important consequence of regional and racial economic inequalities in Brazil has been a massive influx of migrants from rural to urban areas. Over the past 20 years, cities throughout Brazil have absorbed more than 29 million migrants seeking employment and a better life for themselves and their families. Others were evicted from their land by mining projects or cattle raising (International Child Resource Institute 1994). This influx of migrants created a seemingly inexhaustible pool of unskilled laborers in Brazil's large cities. Moreover, the infrastructure of these urban areas has increasingly been unable to expand to meet the demands for health care, education, and employment. As a result, slum dwellings, unemployment, hunger, and violence have risen dramatically. Currently, 75 percent of all Brazilians live in cities, and among them are 52 million boys and girls under age 19 (Eisenstein 1992). This concentration of people in urban areas, combined with poverty and limited health services has placed many segments of the Brazilian population at high risk for epidemic diseases, including HIV/AIDS.

The Sexual Culture of Brazil

Most interpretations of sexuality in Brazil are based on the work of Columbia University's Richard Parker, whose extended field studies of sexual life in Brazil have established the contours of Brazilian sexual culture (Parker 1986, 1991, 1999). Parker's analysis of Brazilian sexual culture is influenced by a social constructionist framework and is sympathetic to French philosopher Michel Foucault's (1978) deconstruction of Western categories of heterosexuality and homosexuality. In Foucault's work, as in Parker's, the focus of inquiry is on the social construction of categories

surrounding a multiplicity of sexual practices. Foucault, for example, examines the emergence of the category "homosexual" in Western nations
and suggests that the act of categorizing sexual practices and desires is a
political one that has serious implications for how people come to organize their desires, their identities, and their relationships with others. In
Western nations, of course, sexuality is defined in terms of three categories: heterosexuality, homosexuality, and bisexuality. To a large extent,
it is believed that erotic desires are relatively fixed throughout one's life
(i.e., women who are sexually attracted to men will not experience sexual
attraction for women), and form a key component of one's identity (i.e.,
having sex and/or desiring a person of the opposite gender establishes
one's heterosexuality, while desiring a person of the same gender establishes one's homosexuality). Subsequently, in most Western nations, categories for locating and understanding sexuality are configured based on
the gender of the person's sexual partners. The object of desire takes
precedence over actual sexual practice in the formation of the categories
homosexual, bisexual, and heterosexual.

Social constructionists argue that constructions of sexuality—
categories of understanding sexual practice—vary among nations, cultures, classes, and subcultures. Parker's exploration of Brazilian sexual
culture is interesting precisely because he uncovers the mutability of sexual categories—that is, our categories for understanding sexuality are
culturally and historically specific, and are not common to many non-
Western countries. In *Bodies, Pleasures, and Passions*, Parker explores the
universe of sexual meanings in Brazil and discusses how cultural constructions of gender, active/passive, dominance/submission, masculin-
ity/femininity, erotic, and forbidden mesh to form an intricate system of
sexual meanings, desires, and practices. In Parker's work with Herbert
Daniel, *Sexuality, Politics, and AIDS in Brazil*, it is argued that understanding sexual culture in Brazil is a crucial prerequisite to any examination of
the introduction, spread, and prevention of HIV/AIDS among Brazilian
people. This work represents an attempt to apply his theoretical discussion of Brazilian sexual culture to a more practical investigation of the
AIDS phenomenon as it is occurring in Brazil.

Foundations of Sexuality: The Gender Hierarchy

Parker (1986, 1991) argues that a number of social structures influence
sexual culture including the country's patriarchal social past, an early
system of slavery, it's multi-ethnic character, the dominance of the
Catholic Church, and the organization of gender relations. Of these, none
is more influential than the organization of relationships between women
and men. The structure of gender serves as the foundation on which all
sexual claims, desires, and practices are organized. Contemporary rela-

tions between men (*homem*) and women (*mulher*) as well as understandings of masculinity (*masculinidade*) and femininity (*femininidade*) are constructed in part from the dichotomy between dominance and submission—a legacy of the country's history of patriarchy.

During the colonial period, the familial social unit consisted of the patriarch, his wife, their children, and a set of mistresses, illegitimate children, slaves, and tenant farmers. Roles among all sets of individuals followed from a strict hierarchy in which the patriarch represented absolute authority—an authority that was based almost entirely on his right to exercise violence. This set of relations was articulated according to the oppositional images of male and female. Men and women were defined in terms of their opposition—men were superior, strong, virile, violent while women were inferior, weak, desirable, and subject to absolute domination by the patriarch. Daily life, too, was divided into oppositional domains of masculine and feminine. Men had absolute sexual freedom and spent most of their day in the public sphere possessing economic, political, and social power. Women's activities, on the other hand, were sharply regulated by the patriarch and were largely confined to the private sphere of household and children. Central to the entire system was the sexual fidelity and chastity of wives and daughters. While women were considered weak and inferior, they retained the capacity to subvert the authority of the patriarch through their sexual infidelities. A man who could not control the sexuality of his wife and daughters was considered weak. Subsequently, women were regarded as potentially dangerous for despite their inferiority, they alone could bring the social downfall of the men who "owned" them.

The historical legacy of patriarchy and the hierarchy between men and women endures into the present day. The oppositional character between masculinity and femininity is reflected in the contemporary language of the body. Parker suggests that the opposition between men and women is embodied in Brazilians' descriptions of the penis and vagina. The penis is frequently referred to as *pau* (stick), *cacete* (club), *pica* (prick—to prick or pierce), *arma* (weapon), *faca* (knife), *bicho* (animal), and *cobra* (snake). The images generated from this vocabulary of the penis are steeped in notions of action, particularly aggressive, violent action. The image of the aggressive penis is made even more explicit by the term *porrada* (beating), which is also used to refer to sex. The term *porra* (verbal rebuke) is also used to describe sperm.

The language of the vagina suggests that it is the object of violence, as well as serving as a place of potential danger. Expressions for the vagina include: *boceta* (box), *buraco* (hole), *chochota* (to become dry, weak), *carne mijada* (meat covered with urine), *boca mijada* (mouth filled with urine), and *aranha* (spider). Parker suggests that tied with the notion of the vagina are symbols of impurity. As the site of menstruation and the flow of waste products, the vagina often comes to stand for uncleanliness, pollution, and contamination.

The language that refers to the penis and vagina serves as the basis for the strict division between masculine and feminine. Central to this opposition is the distinction between active and passive that is embodied in descriptions of the penis and the vagina. *Atividade* (active) and *passividade* (passive) are the most basic categories Brazilians use to organize the sexual universe—these terms come to distinguish men from women, dominance from submission, and masculine from feminine. The language of intercourse—*comer* (to eat), *vencer* (to conquer), *possuir* (to possess), *dar* (to give), *foder* (to fuck)—describe penetration as an act of control and domination.

Despite the stark opposition between masculinity and femininity, there are more than two roles (*homem, mulher*) that take on significance in the Brazilian universe. Masculinity exists not just in opposition to femininity, but in opposition to certain social categories or classes of men including the *machão* (macho), *corno* (cuckold), and *bicha* or *viado* (queer or faggot). Femininity is similarly constructed in opposition to masculinity but with reference to several social categories of women including the *virgem* (virgin), *piranha* or *puta* (whore), and *sapatão* (literally "big shoes" or dyke).

The *machão*, of course, is central to the Brazilian definition of masculinity since it embodies the characteristics of the male role—force, power, violence, aggression, virility, and sexual potency. Just as important for the standard of masculinity, though, are those biological men who fail to live up to it—the *corno* and *bicha*. These social types are instances of a failed masculinity, something that a "true man" can never be. They, like the *machão*, set the perimeters within which all men must model their behavior and identities. *Viado* or *bicha* (literally "worm") refers to men who are believed to take the passive role in sex, that of the penetrated rather than penetrator. As mentioned previously, the distinction between active and passive serves as the central category for organizing sexual relations in Brazil. Because active is definitive of the male role, men who assume a passive role in sexual relations are a cultural anomaly—their masculine anatomy distinguishes them from women yet their preference to be penetrated violates the most basic code of Brazilian masculinity.

Brazilians have handled this apparently anomalous social category by elevating the *viado* to the status of symbolic female. Here, the active/passive model for male-female sexual relations is also used to standardize same-sex contacts between men. Men who maintain the active, penetrator role in same-sex contacts retain their masculine (and ultimately heterosexual) identity. Men who assume the passive role are emasculated and are referred to as being essentially feminine. The *corno*, on the other hand, can be thought of as a castrated male. It refers to men who are unable to control the sexuality of their wives and daughters. He is thought to be weak, like the *viado*, because he can neither satisfy nor control his women.

Like the *homem*, the ideal type of *mulher* is arranged around categories of female roles in Brazil society. For women, the *virgem* is the basis for evaluating and constructing one's femininity. The virgin is defined solely based on her lack of sexual experience, innocence, and her intact hymen. The unbroken hymen serves as testimony to the control her male relatives exercise over her—the hymen marks her innocence as well as the domination of men. Upon marriage, the breaking of the hymen symbolizes the transfer of control of her sexuality from father to husband. To a large extent, women maintain the essential innocence that characterizes the *virgem* even after they have had sex—provided that the initial act (as well as all subsequent acts) occur within the context of their marriage. Because of the centrality of the virgin to male authority, the sexual status of young women is the subject of constant speculation, evaluation, and surveillance. The *puta* (whore) also takes on a central role in the construction of Brazilian femininity. The *puta*, like the *viado*, is an ambiguous figure since her sexual availability confirms the virility and prowess of her male partners, yet at the same time her sexual availability demonstrates the loss of control by her father and brothers. Since the *puta* confirms the virility of her clients, men who have sex with her do not jeopardize their masculinity. On the other hand, she emasculates the men in her family, making them cuckolds. The final social category of women, the *sapatão* or dyke, is the most threatening for femininity since she renounces the basis on which the entire sex/gender system is built. The terms that refer to lesbians—*bota* (boot), *machona* (macho woman), *mulher aranha* (spider woman), and *mulher homem* (man woman)—refer almost exclusively to her supposedly masculine character. Parker notes that the *sapatão* is defined by her masculine character rather than the active/passive role that she assumes in sex (as opposed to the *viado* who is defined by his passive role). He argues, "the very idea of female sexual conduct outside of a context which is in some way or another defined vis-a-vis male sexuality is almost unthinkable in traditional Brazilian life" (Parker 1991:53).

Sexual Socialization

The categories of masculinity and femininity serve as the basis for sexual socialization throughout the life-course, though particularly so during the formative years of early childhood and adolescence. Socialization is the process where the categories dominance/submission, active/passive, and masculinity/femininity are internalized and ultimately performed. Throughout their childhood both boys and girls remain in the feminine sphere of the household and are always in the company of their mother or other appropriate female substitute. For girls, the transition to adulthood is relatively unproblematic as they remain in the female sphere throughout most of their lives and model their behavior after other women in their company. Since the virginity of a daughter is a reflection of the masculine authority of male relatives, girls, particularly upon the onset of their first menstruation, are carefully controlled and guarded. Their freedom of movement is extremely limited and although they begin courting boys at a young age, they are constantly surveilled by adults and peers.

For boys, the emergence into adulthood is more problematic. Because they spend their early years in almost exclusive company of women, boys are confronted by the stigma associated with everything feminine. From the time a boy turns five or six years of age, male relatives begin to chastise him for behaving in a feminine manner. Throughout the rest of his adolescence, boys spend increasing amounts of time in the company of other males and learn that they must define themselves in opposition to everything that is feminine. Often, the process of male sexual socialization is accomplished through older male relatives making pornographic magazines and movies available to adolescent boys. Additionally, many young men have their first sexual experience with a prostitute at their father's behest. Unlike maturing girls, boys are encouraged and often incited by male relatives and peers to lose their virginity because doing so demonstrates their virility and first true accomplishment of masculinity.

Religion and "Acceptable" Sex

Brazilian sexuality is also shaped, in part, by Catholicism and the impact this ideology has on the structure of male domination, female virginity, and sexual practice. Parker argues that Brazilians adopted the "sensual" variant of Catholicism as practiced by the Portuguese and characterized by festivals, feasts, saints who offered advice about love, and a relaxed sexual morality. Within Brazilian Catholicism, a fundamental distinction exists between sexual acts and relations that are legitimate and those that are illegitimate. Sexual conduct that involves marriage, monogamy, and procreation is legitimate, while sexual acts occurring outside these bounds is sinful. Parker suggests that the notion that certain forms of sex are sinful strengthens images of sex as dangerous, polluting, and potentially evil. He argues that an inherent tension exists between religious morality and the gender hierarchy in that demonstrating one's virility often means violating the standards of acceptable sex. While clearly religion does not supplant the gender hierarchy in terms of ordering sexual relationships, it does infuse sexual acts and relations with an added dimension of symbolic meaning and imagery.

The Ideology of the Erotic

Among other structures for understanding the sexual universe in Brazil, Parker argues that there exists another cultural frame—the ideology of the erotic—which is organized differently from other meaning systems in that it is not concerned with hierarchy or encoded moralities, but with an exploration of the diversity of sexual pleasures and practices. Central to organizing the erotic is the notion of transgression and prohibition. The act of categorizing certain sexual practices as illicit or sinful is itself an enticement. Here the oft repeated phrase *"entre quatro paredes, tudo pode acontecer"* (within four walls anything can happen) is salient because it demonstrates the importance of the private realm in organizing sexual experience. What is hidden from public view becomes enticing, seductive—offering the possibility of transgressing certain boundaries without fear of public knowledge and admonishment. *Sacanagem* (trickery, to have sex, or in English, to get fucked over) denotes the range of sexual practices that occur in private—the word itself is often used to imply both aggression, amusement, play, excitement, and sexual practice. In essence, the realm of private sexual experience exists to break the rules of daily life and to transgress sexual boundaries. Subsequently, boundaries such as active/passive, domination/submission, virginity/virility are potentially transgressed in the private realm. Here, no category or prohibition is immutable.

What structures the experience of the erotic in Brazil is determined both by desire and fantasy and a fascination with regions of the body— particularly genitals, but also the mouth, women's breasts, and the anus. Within one's fantasies and desires, anything is possible, one's fascinations with bodies and pleasures can be explored and acted on. The ideology of the erotic places another layer of meaning over images associated with the genitals and the mouth. The penis may be referred to as a weapon, but also as a popsicle, subverting the image of it as something aggressive and conquering. Indeed, images of food, hunger, and eating dominate erotic ideology and language. The traditional gender hierarchy is momentarily suspended when a women has sex on top with a man— she becomes the "active" partner in that she is perceived as "eating" him with her vagina.

While practices such as anal intercourse, masturbation, bisexuality, and homosexuality are considered illegitimate by other meaning structures, in the ideology of the erotic these practices are awarded positive value precisely because they are prohibited. Masturbation, for example, is linked to fantasy and (sexual) indulgence. It can often be tied to a range of homoerotic connotations, in that same-sex settings are not infrequently the site of masturbatory practice. Oral sex, in some cases more so than masturbation, can also serve as an important site for same-sex exchanges, particularly during adolescence. Heterosexual adolescent couples can use this practice to avoid pregnancy and maintain virginity, while same-sex couples use oral sex to explore erotic notions of the tongue, mouth, and genitals. Anal sex, particularly among adolescents, is another common experience. It often becomes a game in which partners take turns playing passive and active roles and maintaining an egalitarian relationship. One saying, "homem, para ser homem, tem que dar primeiro" (a man, in order to be a man, has to give [take passive sexual role] first), demonstrates that older men also frequently participate in anal sex with adolescent boys. Within the world of the erotic, a multiplicity of sexual activities and partners are desired and acted out. These practices extend the range of sexual activities from vaginal sex to include same-sex contacts, anal and oral sex, and singular and mutual masturbation.

"Carnaval" and Sexual Ideology

Carnival in Rio de Janeiro is among the world's wildest, most frantic, and longest party, propelled by a relentless samba beat in the tropical heat of the Brazilian summer. Compared with Carnival, New Orleans's Mardi Gras and Key West's "Fantasy Fest" are like a night at the bowling alley. And Carnival, or "Carnaval" as it is called in Brazil, is celebrated not only in Rio, but throughout the country.

The ideology of the erotic in Brazil can be seen as linked to the ritual of Carnival. In the world of the erotic, that which is prohibited is pursued and acted out. Carnival, an annual three day pre-Lenten festival, is a ritual of reversal in that every form of pleasure is possible—there are no prohibitions that temper sexual practice or desire. It is a time when Brazilians momentarily suspend their moral categories and undertake "dangerous," prohibited practices. In this way, Carnival momentarily serves to both suspend and challenge dominant social structures like religion and the gender hierarchy. Richard Parker argues that in Brazil, sexualities—practices, desires, fantasies—are multiple, abundant, and at times contradictory. Like the ritual of Carnival, erotic ideology and sexual practice thrives on the subversion of social categories and moral prohibitions. To speak of the sexual culture in Brazil is to refer to a sexual terrain that is best characterized by its multiple, shifting, sensuous, and contradictory character—a terrain where the tension between rule and transgression serves as the basis for erotic desire.

Cocaine and Other Drugs in Brazil

Drug use and its consequences are growing concerns throughout much of Brazil. In recent years there have been significant increases in the rates of abuse and dependence on both licit and illicit drugs, and the prevalence of drug use among younger segments of the population has continued to climb (Guerra de Andrade 1995).

The Epidemiology of Drug Use

One of the major obstacles for addressing the drug problem in Brazil is the lack of reliable prevalence statistics that document the scope of drug use within the general population, particularly among adults. Somewhat better data have been collected and compiled by CEBRID (Brazilian Center for Drug Information) on adolescent populations. For example, school surveys showed that in 1993, 17.3 percent of high school students had used illegal drugs at least once in their lifetimes. Among street children, the lifetime prevalence of illegal drug use climbs to between 50.7 percent and 90.5 percent, depending on the city in which they reside.

Other organizations, such as the Narcotics Council of the Federal District of Brasília, have also documented extensive drug use among Brazilian adolescents. The most prevalent drug in Brazil by far is alcohol, as Brazil is the world's largest producer of distilled alcoholic beverages. Perhaps not surprisingly, in a study of 2,100 students in the Brasília area, primarily between the ages of 13 and 18, 17 percent reported drinking alcohol weekly, and 19 percent monthly. In terms of illegal drugs, 10.9 percent had used illegal drugs at least once in their lifetimes, usually beginning between 10 and 15 years of age. Inhalant use had the highest prevalence (11.45%), followed by marijuana (4.95%), and amphetamines (1.4%). Cocaine use was reported by .4 percent and crack by .55 percent (Conselho de Entorpecentes do Distrito Federal 1995).

More recently, prevalence studies of drug-involved adults have begun to document extensive illicit drug use in these populations as well. Drug histories obtained from 294 cocaine users (mean age = 27) attending any of 15 drug treatment agencies in São Paulo during 1996 and 1997 documented that 72 percent were current alcohol users (Dunn et al. 1999). Other lifetime prevalences included: cannabis (96%), solvents (54%), amphetamines (24%), and tranquilizers (51%). Initiation into drug use tended to begin with alcohol use at age 15, followed by cannabis and solvents at age 15.1 or 15.2, amphetamines at age 17.6, cocaine at age 18.9, and tranquilizers at age 22.3. Cocaine was snorted by 87 percent of the sample, smoked by 7 percent, and injected by 6 percent. Only three individuals reported ever using heroin and only two had bought it in Brazil.

A study of 1,544 adult, indigent out-of-treatment cocaine users conducted in Rio de Janeiro found very high lifetime drug use prevalences: 100 percent had used powder cocaine, 97.9 percent had used alcohol, 84.8 percent ever used marijuana, 11.4 percent ever used crack, 1.2 percent ever used heroin, 7.5 percent ever used amphetamines, 2.1 percent ever used inhalants, and 3.8 percent ever used LSD or other hallucinogens. Prevalence in the thirty days prior to interview were also significant: 100 percent currently used powder cocaine, 90.1 percent currently used alcohol, 58.8 percent currently used marijuana, 2.3 percent currently used crack, .1 percent currently used heroin, .8 percent currently used amphetamines, and 2.2 percent currently used any other illegal drug (Surratt and Telles 1999).

Some of Brazil's neighbor nations, especially Colombia, Peru, and Bolivia, have been major producers of cocaine for many years, and cocaine has become an important base of their economies. Brazil has traditionally occupied the role of a transit point (especially in the Amazon region), and has been a consumer country, especially in the large, important cities (Guerra de Andrade 1995). As a result, cities along the cocaine trafficking routes from Bolivia to São Paulo and Rio de Janeiro have been plagued with many of the consequences of drug use, especially violence and AIDS (Fagundes 1997). Injection drug use is common in these cities, and drug injectors comprise the majority of the AIDS cases in these locales. In fact, they have on average twice the number of AIDS cases as cities with similar population profiles located off the cocaine transit route, and they have four times the number of AIDS cases among injection drug users.

Crack Cocaine

Crack cocaine first appeared in Brazil on the streets of São Paulo in 1988 (Uchôa 1996). Exactly who was responsible for introducing crack remains a mystery, however, but it quickly became popular and began to rival *powder* cocaine as the most sought after drug in the city. Because the average price for a crack "rock" is R$10 (U.S.$6 to $10 depending on Brazilian currency fluctuations), crack was accessible to a wide range of users, particularly the young and the poor. One indication of crack's popularity in São Paulo is that of the 5,000 drug-selling points in the city, 80 percent sell only crack (Uchôa 1996), and police estimate that there are more than 150,000 crack users in metropolitan São Paulo alone.

Rio de Janeiro seems to be the only large city in Brazil where crack cocaine is not easily available. Although there is no clear explanation for this pattern of distribution, anecdotal reports suggest that the two main trafficking organizations in Rio de Janeiro, the Comando Vermelho (Red Command) and the Terceiro Comando (Third Command) seem to control almost all drug commerce in the city, and that the drug trade is clearly more organized in Rio de Janeiro than in other major cities. This situation is unique to Rio de Janeiro, and in other cities the drug trade is less localized, apparently scattered between various small gangs or isolated individuals. As a consequence, the trade is less affected by the decisions or rules dictated by a specific organization. In Rio de Janeiro, crack cocaine, also known as *paulista exótico* because of its association with São Paulo, seems to be repudiated by the local traffickers. One trafficker in the Morro do Dendê, who controls 60 soldiers and sells more than 140 kilos of marijuana and powder cocaine per month explained:

> Here we only have "rice and beans." Cocaine and marijuana. Everything is high quality. There is no selling rocks. What is the deal with that? Here rocks are only for building houses, repairing shacks. Crack has not arrived in Rio and is never going to arrive because there is no market for it. We will not let that drug come into the *favela*. You may have people below that are messing around with it and making it, but what they do with the powder after they buy it here doesn't concern me. But they will not smoke it here. This is a job like any other. When an employee starts to make mistakes what does the boss do? He reprimands him or sends him packing. Here it is the same thing. Our soldiers are people we have to trust. They stay in line. They have schedules, earn salaries and everything. It is like a business. If someone shows up with a rock, they have to go. There is no second chance. How can I trust a soldier that smokes crack? The guy gets so out of it that his mind is not on his work. Bad employees are out on the street. Here this is the law (Uchôa 1996:84).

Police officials concur that crack has entered neither the city nor the state of Rio de Janeiro because the trafficking culture is well organized. Destitute people, living in shantytowns, obey the commands of the local leaders. They live in marginal areas essentially without government, so they rely on the traffickers to provide for them and in return they respect their authority. Crack is seen by these leaders as an evil drug.

HIV/AIDS in Brazil

To a considerable extent, HIV and AIDS in Brazil have been dominated by Western medical discourse regarding sexual practice and epidemiological patterns. This, combined with homophobia, poverty and inequality, cocaine, and limited health care resources, has resulted in the failure of Brazilian public policy and medical technology to adequately address the disease.

Brazil became aware of the AIDS epidemic in the early 1980s from media accounts of the disease in Western nations, particularly the United States. Based on those reports and the dominance of Western "sexual preference" designations of heterosexual and homosexual, AIDS was believed to be a disease that targeted wealthy, promiscuous, gay men. By 1986, the epidemiological patterns of the disease in Brazil were radically different from the images that had been generated by early reports, but it was this early portrait that continued to serve as the basis for the government's questionable response. Indeed, while most AIDS cases were located in urban areas, AIDS had spread to every region in the country and was increasingly penetrating indigent sectors of society. Further, by 1991, the spread of the disease through heterosexual contact and injection drug use rose dramatically making this a disease that could no longer be considered to be confined exclusively to gay and bisexual men.

Using Western paradigms of sexual practice and AIDS transmission has generated a number of problems for Brazilians attempting to stave off the spread of HIV and AIDS. First, Western categories of "homosexual" and "heterosexual" are not synonymous with Brazilian categories of *viado* and *machão* (Parker 1991, 1999). As noted earlier, men who maintain an active (penetrator) role in same-sex relations do not categorize themselves as gay or bisexual. Early media reports and government public service announcements that targeted "homosexuals" obscured the fact that certain sexual practices (rather than categories of persons) were a significant vectors for transmission of the virus. Second, the lack of a significant, clearly defined gay community in Brazil resulted in minimal political activism or community mobilization among the persons most afflicted. Small sexual subcultures do exist in such larger cities as Rio de Janeiro, São Paulo, Belo Horizonte, and Porto Alegre, but these are organized more around divergent sexual practices and less around issues of "gay" identity as is the case in the United States. Third, Brazil was unprepared for the unprecedented number of AIDS cases that emerged from blood transfusions. Unlike Western nations, there was a lack of regulation over the exchange of blood, and a number of clandestine blood banks existed to profit from blood sales (whose donors are generally from the poorest classes). Fortunately, the Brazilian government has more recently increased and enforced blood screening regulations so that the country's blood supply is now protected against HIV. Finally, like many industrialized nations, including the United States, Brazil has treated injection drug use as a legal rather than as a medical problem. This delayed such prevention, intervention, and harm reduction activities as needle exchange and bleach disinfection programs from being mobilized on a national basis (see Epilogue). And finally, because of the issues of poverty, inequality, and the designation of *favela* residents as "disposable," HIV prevention/intervention/outreach programs into their communities were not considered a priority.

Postscript

Sexual practices in Brazil are multiple, fluid, and shifting. Dominating the sexual landscape are the categories active/passive and prohibition/transgression. The apparent popularity of anal sex and same-sex contacts bring a whole new set of implications for understanding the spread of AIDS in Brazil among both gays and heterosexuals. It is not uncommon for *machão* men to have sex with their wives, mistresses, female prostitutes, male prostitutes, and *travestis*—male transvestite sex workers (see Chapter 6). Further, because of the importance of prohibition and transgression, sexual practices vary—men may engage in anal sex with women, they may be the passive recipients of anal sex from other men, or they may be the active or passive recipients of anal and oral sex with transvestites.

The economy of sex in Brazil also has a number of implications for the spread of HIV/AIDS. Contrary to public notions, it is male prostitutes and transvestites—not female prostitutes—who appear to have higher rates of HIV infection. Indeed, a unique subculture has emerged around the occupation of male sex worker. Male sex workers are divided into *miches* ("hypermasculine" men who are believed to assume an active role in sexual relations with a predominantly gay client base), and *travestis* (men who take on feminine characteristics and assume primarily passive roles). *Miches* often come from poorer segments of Brazilian society and typically service more well-to-do clients. Many *miches* continue to live with their families and engage in heterosexual relations with women. The *travestis* are also drawn from lower classes, but because of their feminine characteristics, they are usually forced to leave home and relocate in subcultural enclaves in the cities. And there is a significant market for the services of the *travestis* (see Chapter 6). Most clients of the *travestis* do not consider themselves gay because of the fact that the *travestis* are considered as symbolic females despite the nature of the sexual acts that are performed.

Notes

1. Because Brazilian currency tends to change and/or lose value rapidly, income is frequently calculated in terms of the number of minimum salaries earned, rather than a fixed monetary value. At the close of 1996, the minimum wage per month was R$100, or $93.00 in U.S. currency.

3

Establishing an
HIV/AIDS Intervention Program in
a Developing Nation

By the beginning of 1999, Brazil had reported almost 165,000 documented cases of AIDS to the World Health Organization (Brazilian Ministry of Health 1999). As such, Brazil has the second largest number of known AIDS cases in the world, surpassed only by the United States (WHO 1999). In addition to these confirmed cases of AIDS, toward the close of 1999 the Brazilian Ministry of Health reported that there were at least 536,000 persons living with HIV infection, with the majority in the heavily populated southeastern part of the country (Brazilian Ministry of Health 1999).

The initial cases of AIDS in Brazil were identified in 1982 in the states of Rio de Janeiro and São Paulo, where one and four cases were recorded, respectively (Rodrigues and Chequer 1989). In 1983, 31 more cases were recognized, with notable increases in subsequent years. By the 1990s, the annual incidence rates per hundred thousand population had increased significantly, from .05 in 1982 to 5.9 in 1990, to 11.0 in 1993, and to 12.2 in 1999 (Brazilian Ministry of Health 1995, 1999).

The highest concentrations of AIDS cases have occurred in the southeastern region of the country, in the cities of São Paulo (22.5%) and Rio de Janeiro (10.0%), and among those in the 25- to 40- year-old age group (59.7%). As illustrated in Figures 3.1 and 3.2, sexual transmission accounts for the majority of cases, followed by injection drug use, other/unknown cause, blood transfusions, perinatal, and hemophiliac. The actual number of AIDS cases in Brazil is likely grossly underestimated, given diagnostic deficiencies and the prevailing social climate, which reflects a generalized (and sometimes quite specific) discrimination against people with AIDS (Quinn et al. 1990; Zacarais 1990; Daniel and Parker 1993).

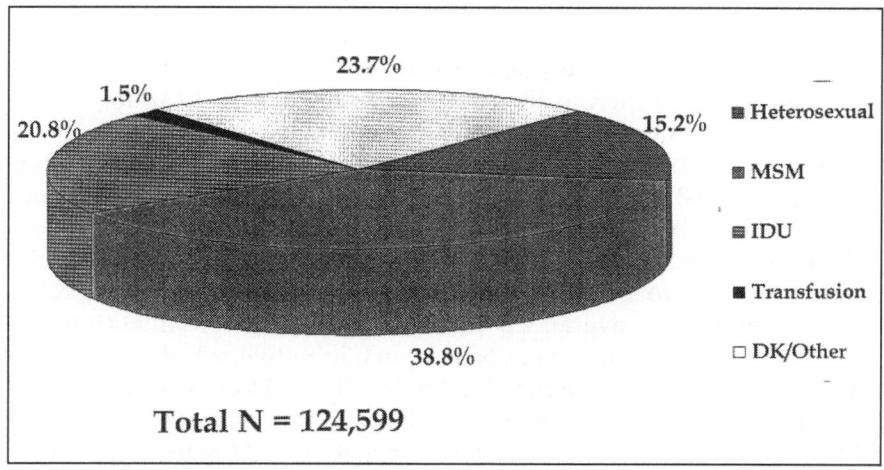

FIGURE 3.1   Distribution of AIDS Cases in Brazil by Exposure Category, Males, 1980–1999.

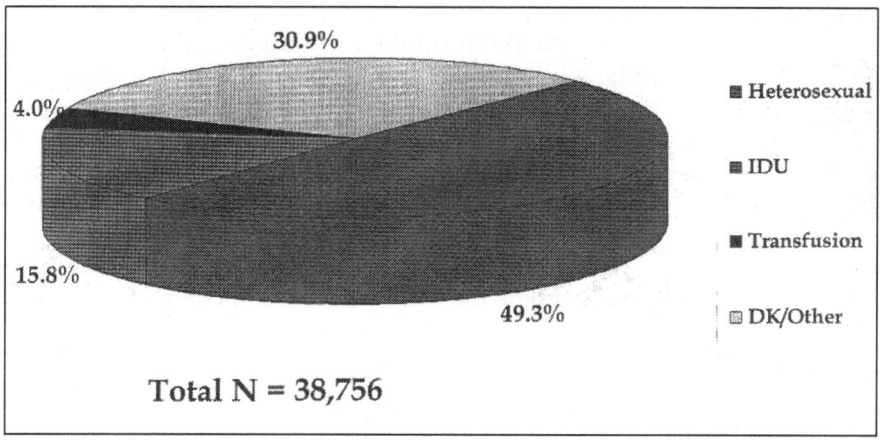

FIGURE 3.2   Distribution of AIDS Cases in Brazil by Exposure Category, Females, 1980–1999.

Numerous early studies suggested that rates of HIV infection were considerably high in Rio de Janeiro among injection drug users, heterosexual partners of male bisexuals, transfusion recipients, and male and female prostitutes (Telles et al. 1992; Guimarães et al. 1991; Cortes et al. 1989a, 1989b). And more recently, in a study of 699 injection drug users recruited from street locations in Rio de Janeiro and Santos, 33 percent and 63 percent, respectively, tested positive for HIV (Telles et al. 1994). Independent risk factors for HIV infection among these drug users included (1) more than five years of injection drug use, (2) being a man who had sex with men in the previous five years, and (3) not having taken deliberate steps to protect oneself from infection.

Recognizing the critical need to address the growing problem of AIDS in Brazil, in 1993 the Community Research Branch of the National Institute on Drug Abuse (NIDA) funded a research demonstration prevention/intervention initiative targeting segments of Rio de Janeiro populations at high risk for HIV/AIDS acquisition and transmission. The project was part of NIDA's overall Cooperative Agreement for AIDS Community-Based Outreach/Intervention Research initiative, which included 23 sites ranging from Anchorage, Alaska, to Miami, Florida, and from San Juan, Puerto Rico, to Rio de Janeiro, Brazil (see Figure 3.3). The overall NIDA cooperative agreement initiative began in 1990 with the purposes of (1) preventing the further spread of HIV/AIDS among injection and other drug users, (2) sampling and monitoring the serostatus of these populations, and (3) evaluating the efficacy of controlled experimental interventions designed to eliminate or reduce HIV risk behaviors (Inciardi and Needle 1998).

The Cooperative Agreement effort had a set of protocols that applied to all of its 23 projects, with only minor variations from site to site. The research process conformed with the following general procedures:

- Target populations included injection drug users and crack smokers (and in Rio de Janeiro, cocaine injectors and snorters). Eligible cases had to be at least 18 years of age, had to have used illegal drugs (injected/smoked/snorted) in the past 30 days, and be out of treatment for the last 30 days. There had to be verification of drug use through examination for needle marks/tracks and/or a positive drug test.
- Clients were recruited by indigenous outreach workers through "targeted sampling" (Watters and Biernacki 1989) and "chain referral" (Inciardi 1986) strategies in specific geographic locales where drug use rates were high.
- Outreach was a proactive process in which workers engaged potential clients in a screening process and a preliminary discussion of AIDS prevention. Hygiene kits were distributed that contained condoms, needle cleaning equipment, AIDS prevention literature (including how to use a condom and how to clean injection equipment), and referral information for sexually transmitted disease (STD) testing and drug abuse treatment.

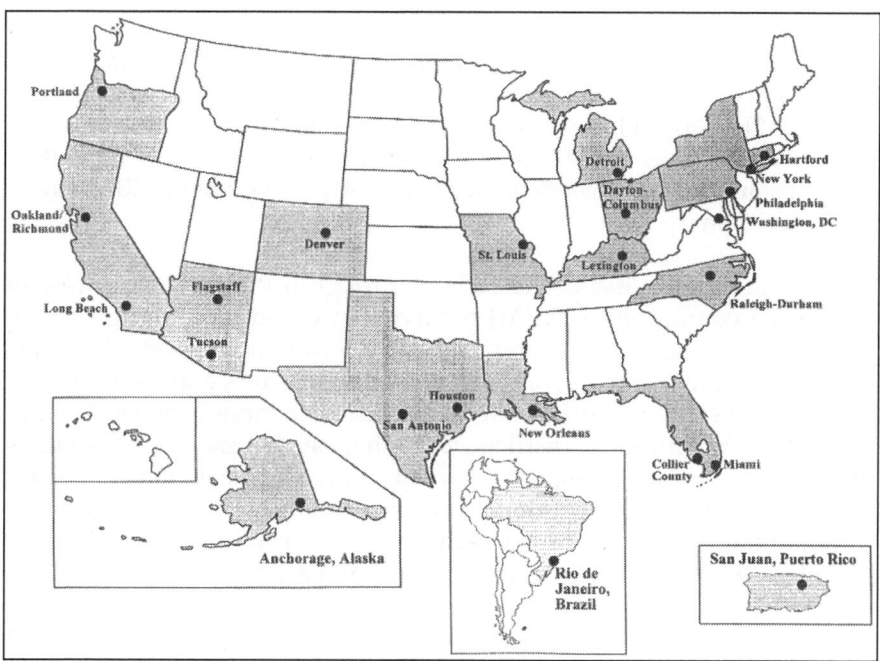

FIGURE 3.3   Cooperative Agreement for AIDS Community-Based Outreach/
Intervention Research Program Sites

- Eligible clients were given an appointment for intake at a project
  site/assessment center. Intake included informed consent, drug
  testing, administration of a standardized "Risk Behavior Assessment" (RBA) instrument and locator form, a recruitment trailer
  form, and site-specific instruments (if any).
- Pretest HIV prevention counseling was provided, covering such
  topics as HIV disease, transmission routes, risky behaviors, risks
  associated with crack or cocaine use, rehearsal of condom use,
  stopping unsafe sex practices, communication with partners,
  cleaning and disinfection of injection equipment, rehearsal of
  needle and syringe cleaning, disposal of hazardous waste material, stopping unsafe drug use, benefits of drug treatment, HIV
  testing, literature and referrals, and distribution of the hygiene
  kits.
- HIV testing was provided to all clients on a voluntary basis.
- Posttest counseling and HIV test results were provided one to
  three weeks after testing.

- At the majority of the Cooperative Agreement sites, there was random assignment of participants either to NIDA's "Standard Intervention" at the pretest counseling phase of the project, or to an "Enhanced Intervention," which varied by site.[1]
- An effort was made to reassess all participants at follow-up with a standardized Risk Behavior Follow-Up Assessment (RBFA) instrument.

The general purposes of the authors' project in Rio de Janeiro were to establish a community HIV/AIDS surveillance and monitoring system, and to develop, implement, and evaluate a community-based HIV/AIDS prevention/intervention program for cocaine injectors and snorters, and male transvestite sex workers, in Rio's hillside shantytowns (*favelas*) and "red light" (prostitution) districts, and other neighborhoods where rates of street drug use were high. A secondary purpose was to develop an effective field-based HIV prevention program that could be used in other communities throughout Brazil and perhaps other developing nations.

Within the context of these introductory remarks, the purposes of this chapter are to (1) examine the steps involved in developing and implementing a complex research project in an international setting, (2) detail the nature of the problems encountered in this project and how they were reckoned with, (3) explore the cultural issues that impacted on project operations, and (4) offer suggestions and insights for other researchers contemplating work in the international sector.

Developing the Research Protocols

For the great majority of investigators who generate research projects in the United States, the initial procedures are fairly clear. After the research questions are conceptualized and a design is assembled, a grant application is prepared, a budget is computed, human subjects protocols are examined by the principal investigator's institutional review board (IRB), and the application is submitted to the appropriate funding agency—generally through the institution at which the principal investigator has his or her primary appointment. The only difficult step in this process is writing an application of merit sufficient to receive a fundable score at peer review. All of the other stages are considered routine and taken for granted. This, however, is not the case with the planning of international research. Even for those investigators who are well seasoned in the grant development and writing process and have contacts at an international site, the planning phase can be quite complex. When the proposal for this project in Brazil was prepared, the principal investigator was quite naive about the intricacies of international work—even after numerous visits to the planned site.

Selecting the Research Site

At the outset, Rio de Janeiro appeared to be an ideal place for establishing an HIV/AIDS prevention/intervention project for injection drug users, for a variety of reasons. First, there appeared to be a major drug problem. Although heroin use was always minimal in Rio (Masur and Cotrim 1987), with the emergence and growth of coca production in the north of Brazil and cocaine trafficking through the north and south since the late 1970s, anecdotal and media reports suggested that the use of *basuco* (coca paste) and powder cocaine (both snorting and injecting) were rather widespread in most of the large urban areas (Rio de Janeiro *O Globo*, 26 July 1987: 22; *O Estado de São Paulo*, 10 November 1990: 5; São Paulo *Veja*, 12 December 1990: 22–23). Furthermore, although school surveys conducted by the State University of Rio de Janeiro in 1980 found that only 3 in every 100 students had either smoked marijuana or sniffed cocaine, by 1991 that proportion had increased to 1 in every 5 (São Paulo *Veja*, 27 March 1991: 42–48). In addition, studies sponsored by the World Health Organization suggested that there were likely more than 30,000 cocaine injectors in Rio de Janeiro (Bastos et al. 1988; Lima et al. 1990). And finally, although crack cocaine was viewed by Brazilians as a U.S. inner-city drug when the principal investigator first visited Brazil in 1989, reports of crack use and crack seizures began appearing regularly since August 1991, primarily in São Paulo (Rio de Janeiro *O Globo*, 23 August 1991: 8; Rio de Janeiro *Jornal do Brasil*, 7 September 1991: 1; São Paulo *O Estado de São Paulo*, 7 September 1991: 17; Rio de Janeiro *O Globo*, 23 September 1991: 10; São Paulo *Visão*, 9 October 1991: 42–43; Rio de Janeiro *Jornal do Brasil*, 24 October 1991: 2).

Second, a variety of small-scale studies also suggested that rates of HIV infection among injection drug users, prostitutes, and men who have sex with men in Rio de Janeiro were significant. For example, of 36 injection drug users tested as part of a larger World Health Organization study in Rio, 33 percent were found to be seropositive (Lima et al. 1991; Lima et al. 1993); of 54 heterosexual partners of male bisexuals and transfusion recipients, 51.8 percent were found to be HIV positive (Guimarães et al. 1991); of 33 male prostitutes (36 percent homosexual and 64 percent bisexual), 43 percent were positive for HIV (Cortes et al. 1989a); of 34 "lower class" female prostitutes from Rio brothels, 9 percent were positive for HIV (Cortes et al. 1989b). As such, it appeared that HIV and AIDS were well established in Rio de Janeiro.

Third, the principal investigator had become well acquainted with substance abuse/AIDS researchers in Rio de Janeiro who had received funding both locally and internationally, and had connections with segments of the drug abuse research community in the United States. As such, everything seemed to be in place for the preparation of a major grant application. However, things were not quite as straightforward as they appeared.

For example, although the published data were sketchy and sometimes anecdotal, *that was all there was*—particularly with respect to drug use. The problem was that little systematic drug abuse research was being conducted in developing nations at that time. What *was* being done was accomplished with limited funds and staffing, and as a result, samples were typically very small and not necessarily representative. Moreover, only a few researchers publish their findings in English language journals, further limiting a U.S.-based researcher's access to data. And finally, because drug abuse research is only a recent enterprise in Brazil (see Monteiro and Inciardi 1993), few investigators have developed a cadre of key informants and street contacts who can provide insights into the community epidemiology of drug abuse.

Because of these obstacles, the principal investigator had numerous discussions with drug abuse researchers in Rio de Janeiro and other Brazilian cities prior to the preparation of the grant application. However, much of the data on which the proposal was based were misleading as far as the project's research design was concerned. As it turned out, and although cocaine use was indeed widespread in Rio de Janeiro, injection drug users—the primary targets of the research—were actually few in number by the time fieldwork actually commenced. Many had been infected with HIV early in the epidemic, and had subsequently died from AIDS prior to the onset of the research. In addition, injection drug users were blamed for much of the spread of AIDS in Rio de Janeiro, and as a result, many had gone into hiding or stopped injecting. And finally, because a good bit of the cocaine sold on the streets of Rio de Janeiro is cut with marble powder, it is difficult to inject. As such, the preferred route of administration of cocaine was, and continues to be, intranasal.

Although the project expanded its sampling frame to include cocaine *snorters*—among whom there also were significant rates of HIV infection—there was a lesson to be learned. Prior to considering a study at an international site, it is imperative that a good understanding of the local drug scene is obtained. If existing research data are not well developed, or if samples are extremely small, pilot study is warranted. At the very least, extensive focus groups with target populations as well as ethnographic data from key informants would appear to be mandatory.

Developing the Budget

Budgets are always a problem, even when dealing with one's own institution's salary arrangement and fringe benefit plan, and one's own country's price structure, economy, inflation rates, and labor laws. However, when dealing with U.S.-based institutions, a few things are systematized: there is a standardized salary structure (or at the very least a framework for one), and a relatively fixed fringe benefit rate. Although one can never be sure about inflation, the prices of supplies, equipment, and services generally remain stable. The biggest difficulty is figuring out actual budgetary needs three, four, or five years into the project. When generating a budget for a project in a developing nation, little of the conventional wisdom applies, particularly with respect to budgets.

When the budget was developed in 1991 for this five-year research project, it was done in Rio de Janeiro, with the help of Brazilian researchers and administrators. Salaries were negotiated with the principal scientists; the costs of recurring items were determined; payments to outreach workers, interviewers, and counselors were estimated; and training and travel costs were projected. Because the budget was based on the U.S. dollar, and since the Brazilian cruzeiro was undergoing triple-digit devaluation at the time, it was believed that all expenses would be covered adequately.

When the project was implemented, however, it was quickly learned that those who were initially consulted with for pricing estimates were unaware of, or had forgotten about, many of the actual and less obvious costs. For example, fringe benefits had been estimated to be 20 percent, when in fact, they were 48 percent according to the system of labor laws under which the project was established. Moreover, a fringe benefit in Brazil is a thirteenth month of salary, paid in December each year. Neither of these had been factored into the budget. Moreover, the principal investigator was not made aware of the fact that in addition to Brazil's 35 paid holidays (and sometimes Fridays when the holiday lands on a Thursday), staff expected to receive five weeks of paid Christmas leave. This had an impact on the availability of staff needed to meet project goals.

Going further, the costs of outreach, interviewing, and counseling had been substantially underestimated. The original plan was to pay the majority of these costs under a per case/piecework basis. In practice, however, staff could not be found who would work under such an arrangement. Similarly, currency exchange charges and bank taxes had not been included in the original budget calculations. In addition, many of the cost estimates for supplies and equipment, as well as overall staffing needs so as to conform to cultural differences and expectations were underestimated.

Ultimately, although the budget that was awarded for the project was not increased, it was restructured to meet all unexpected costs, and the staffing structure was reorganized under an alternative labor agreement so as to reduce the fringe benefit rate somewhat. The price paid, however, was a high one. Much of the Rio-based scientific staff had to be eliminated, with the work shifting to the U.S.-based staff. In addition, to reduce the costs of supplies and equipment, these were purchased in the U.S. and shipped (or carried as "baggage" by the principal investigator and coprincipal investigator) duty-free to Rio de Janeiro under a Brazilian customs regulation that permits the *donation* of goods and materials from foreign organizations to nonprofit institutions in Brazil.

Less than a year into the project, and after more than a decade of devastating inflation, Brazil stabilized its currency and shifted from the beleaguered cruzeiro (Cr$) to the more promising "real" (R$). However, because the value of the new real remained stabilized only because of government supports, the U.S. dollar became extremely weak in Brazil during 1995. And because salaries were based on the dollar, all staff members experienced the equivalent of a 20 percent pay reduction. Not surprisingly, dissatisfactions among the staff emerged.

There were other problems as well, but the point is clear. When developing budgets for research in international settings, a number of things must be done well in advance. Researchers, administrators, and fiscal personnel must be consulted to determine *true* staffing requirements and costs, labor laws, fringe benefits, and other monetary nuances. Local research institutions and projects should be visited for the purpose of better understanding alternative mechanisms for organizing personnel and costs. And finally, since most U.S. funding agencies are not permitted under federal regulations to provide supplements because of inflation, the potential for inflation or currency devaluation should be built into the project at the outset.

Institutional Arrangements

Funds for the great majority of research projects in the United States flow directly from the sponsoring government agency to the grants, contracts, or research administration office of the receiving institution. In most cases, the receiving institution is a college, university, or not-for-profit corporation that has mechanisms in place for the disbursement and monitoring of these research funds. This is not necessarily the case with research in foreign settings.

By contrast, the flow of funds for the Rio-based project was far more complex. The initial arrangement was for funds to move from the National Institute on Drug Abuse (NIDA) to the University of Miami School of Medicine, with a subcontract to Núcleo de Estudos e Pesquisas em Atenção ao Uso de Drogas (NEPAD), a nonprofit drug treatment and research center affiliated with the State University of Rio de Janeiro (UERJ). However, NEPAD researchers indicated that UERJ, and similar institutions, had no research administration units as in the U.S., and that if funds were sent directly to UERJ they might become lost in an administrative "black hole," never to be seen again. The alternative was to have the funds administered through Sociedade de Estudos e Pesquisas em Drogadicção (SEPED)—an incorporated, not-for-profit, professional association affiliated with the university research group.

Although all of that may appear to be fairly straightforward, there were problems—significant problems. For example, U.S. federal regulations do not permit payments of indirect costs to foreign institutions. This caused immediate difficulties, because NEPAD and UERJ had made a number of commitments to the project in anticipation of overhead funds—commitments involving space as well as fiscal and administrative support. After extensive negotiations, NEPAD donated eight rooms to the project, while the project paid for the actual costs incurred by NEPAD to administer the project.

The more difficult and cumbersome problem related to cash flow and ,hence, payroll and other payments in Brazil. Unlike most U.S.-based research institutions that have enough cash on hand to operate on a cost-reimbursable basis, this is not the case with many institutions in developing nations. The University of Miami, on the other hand, was reluctant to advance large sums of money to an organization in South America with which it had never had prior dealings. Moreover, even if Miami had been willing, it had no institutionalized mechanism to do so.

A system was established that, in theory, appeared workable. But as "Murphy's Law" often dictates, many things went wrong, particularly since bureaucratic entanglements are endemic with "accounts payable" and "accounts receivable" units in universities around the world. In consequence, sometimes checks failed to arrive on time, and the payment of bills and salaries had to be delayed. Not surprisingly, this situation had an impact on staff morale.

What can be learned from the situation is this. When an investigator is contemplating international research, the payment procedures should be negotiated and established in advance. Moreover, such negotiations should take place with both the sending and receiving institutions, and letters of agreement that succinctly detail the steps in the payment process should be signed by the principal investigator and the fiscal officers of the all of the institutions involved.

Human Subjects and Other Clearances

Potential investigators should understand that although an international project may have been approved both for scientific merit and for agency funding, an actual award notice may be considerably delayed pending a wide variety of clearances. These authorizations are of both domestic and international origin.

The Office for Protection from Research Risks (OPRR) at the National Institutes of Health, for example, has a complex and lengthy set of instructions and requirements so as to assure that human subjects are adequately protected. Most institutions in the United States participating in research with human subjects have been granted a "Multiple Project Assurance" (MPA) from OPRR. This means that a "master document" has been filed with, and approved by, OPRR that guarantees that all federal regulations associated with the protection of human subjects against research risks will be adhered to. It also means that the institution has a standing Institutional Review Board (IRB)—a committee of scientists who meet regularly to review research grant applications for the purpose of determining whether human subjects will be adequately protected.

Because the University of Miami School of Medicine has an MPA from OPRR as well as an IRB that reviewed the project's human subjects protocol, it was believed that there would be no "human subjects" problems. Moreover, the peer review committee at NIDA that evaluated the grant application determined that human subjects would not be at risk. As such, it was presumed that the "human subjects" issue was settled. However, this was an incorrect assumption. Because the State University of Rio de Janeiro (UERJ) was the subcontractor that would be conducting the outreach, interviewing, urine and HIV testing, and pretest and posttest counseling, it too was required to meet OPRR protocols. Yet it had neither an MPA nor an IRB. As a solution, UERJ filed a "Single Project Assurance" with OPRR. However, this turned out to be a complex task because UERJ had no IRB of its own. One was finally found at the Rio de Janeiro State Narcotics Council, and that organization assumed responsibility for the protection of human subjects.

Other clearances had to come from the Brazilian Ministry of Health, the Brazilian Ministry of Foreign Affairs, the U.S. Embassy in Brasília, the U.S. Consulate in Rio de Janeiro, and the United States Department of State in Washington, D.C. And since the clearances with government officials in Brazil had to be coordinated through the U.S. State Department and the National Institutes of Health, bureaucratic entanglements and jurisdictional issues emerged. All of these clearances delayed project initiation by almost a year, and the point of this discussion is that "start-up" dates must be extremely flexible.

Establishing the Research Site

Researchers in the United States who have studied either "hidden," "street-based," "at risk," "deviant," and/or "criminal" groups are already well aware of the methods and all of the dangers associated with accessing and researching *hidden populations*. Not only are there crime and safety concerns, but in addition there are special staffing considerations. At an international site these factors may take on added significance. Moreover, there are a range of issues associated with language and cultural differences that impact on the overall grant operations.

Crime and Safety Issues

There are many dangerous cities in the world. At different times and for diverse reasons, such urban areas in the U.S. as New York, Miami, Los Angeles, Detroit, New Orleans, and Washington, D.C., to name but a few have been designated as the "crime capitals" or "murder capitals" of the nation. Although these labels are often applied by a pandering and exaggerating mass media, American cities can indeed be dangerous places at times—at least in certain neighborhoods and at particular times of the day (but typically at night). Local researchers generally know the "street scene," and take precautions to ensure their safety, and that of their staff and research site.

The rules are often different with research settings in many developing nations. In Latin America, for example, the concept of "dangerous places" exists at a very different level. Such urban centers as Bogota (Colombia), Caracas (Venezuela), Lima (Peru), and Rio de Janeiro (Brazil) during the 1990s, have indeed been world "murder capitals," and there are numerous others where the hazard quotient is extremely high. What adds to the danger are elements that are not necessarily present in U.S. cities (or not to the same degree)—extreme class differences, very large indigent populations, police corruption and brutality, the survival of military dictatorship ideology, police and citizen "death squads," gross human rights violations, and street warfare. Understandably, all of these impact on street-based research.

In the Rio de Janeiro project, there were some special risks and hazards that brought about several adjustments in the research protocols. Much of the project's client recruitment occurred in several of the 545 *favelas* in which no less than 1 million *cariocas* (residents of Rio de Janeiro) live. The *favelas* (described in greater detail in Chapter 4) are slums in which only a small portion of households have electricity, running water, or sewage facilities. In the absence of public medical facilities and unemployment benefits for the more than 50 percent of the out-of-work *favelados*, disease and social problems multiply. There is prostitution and drug use, and a key feature of most *favelas* is cocaine trafficking (Guillermoprieto 1990).

Street-based cocaine sales are conducted quite differently in Brazilian *favelas* than in America's inner-city drug neighborhoods. For example, just after the initiation of fieldwork in Rio de Janeiro, a visit was made to Mangueira, one of several *favelas* situated in close proximity to the university complex where the project was based, and where client recruitment occurred. Within minutes of entering Mangueira, the investigators happened upon a local cocaine dealer going about his daily business of selling drugs. What was most different about the setting was that the dealer was surrounded by three of his "controllers"—local thugs, high on cocaine, and armed with MAC–10, TEC–9, and KG–9 automatic weapons. Also present were the various "lookouts" (who watch for strangers and the police) and "airplanes" (who take the drugs to the users), who work for the local *traficante* (trafficker). All of this was in plain sight, and almost immediately the investigators were confronted by the controllers, questioning the reasons for their presence. Such a situation makes for difficulties in participant observation, ethnographic mapping, and other forms of fieldwork.

Going further, on several occasions during 1994 and 1995, there was open warfare in several *favelas* between the military and the drug gangs (*Folha de São Paulo*, 3 November 1994:2; São Paulo *Veja*, 2 November 1994:34–37; Rio de Janeiro *O Globo*, 14 November 1994:13). Oftentimes, there were shooting wars between rival *traficantes* (São Paulo *Agência Estado*, 1739 Greenwich Mean Time, 25 January 1995). On all of these occasions, outreach workers had to be brought in from the field and client recruitment suspended.

There were safety issues proximate to the research site as well. Because all of the project's clients were active cocaine users, their presence at the site attracted a variety of individuals of questionable intent. Thus, even though the building in which the project was housed had Rio de Janeiro State security officers, the project nevertheless had to have its own security personnel. In addition, procedures were established to ensure clients from rival *favelas* were not scheduled to visit the project at the same time.

As a result of these and other experiences, the lesson to be learned is clear: crime and security problems must be researched in advance, anticipated, and accounted for in the preparation of an application and the organizing of a research site.

Cultural Differences

In an effort to develop a culturally sensitive grant application, the principal investigator inquired into pertinent differences in the folkways, mores, traditions, and occupational and financial issues that might impact on the overall research effort. Not surprisingly, there were both gaps and disparities in the principal investigator's information. Moreover, there were some problems with the details on cultural issues provided by the Brazilian professionals consulted with prior to the preparation of the application. A major difficulty was that not only the Americans, but also the Brazilians involved in generating the research plan failed to recognize *all* of the cultural differences that would have consequences for the project. Critical in this regard were significant issues associated with staff selection and organization, and work assignments.

First, work assignments in many sectors of employment throughout Brazil are often extremely fragmented and compartmentalized, in that any individual employee has a few very specific tasks rather than a wide range of expectations. For example, in restaurants it is not uncommon to see one employee bringing water, another serving coffee, a third clearing and cleaning tables, a fourth taking orders, and still another serving the food. Before leaving the restaurant, the bill will be prepared by one employee, the amount on the check or credit card slip verified by another, and the cash or credit slip taken by a third. In the U.S., all of these tasks are done by a waiter, or waiter and cashier. Whether this tradition of specificity and compartmentalization is a legacy of the Portuguese colonial administration, Brazilian military rule, or a compromised economic system that resulted in workers having many different part-time jobs, it can have a major impact on a complex research project.

At the HIV intervention project, for example, interviewers were hired to administer two intricate questionnaires—the RBA (Risk Behavior Assessment) and RBFA (Risk Behavior Follow-Up Assessment). A few months into the project, a short field questionnaire was added to the bank of instruments, and the principal investigator and coprincipal investigator could not understand why there was resistance by the interviewers to filling it out. It was a simple, one-page document that would take but a few minutes to complete. Moreover, preparing the additional instrument would not cause added hours or even minutes at work each day, because there was considerable "down time" between interviews. It was quickly learned that the interviewers felt that since they had been hired to administer RBAs and RBFAs, they should not be required to fill out field questionnaires as well. Doing so called for extra pay. This situation emerged several times throughout the project, requiring continual adjustments in the salary structure and deployment of work.

A second staffing situation emerged with respect to outreach activities. The project called for experienced field-workers going into certain target areas where rates of drug use were high, for the purposes of engaging potential clients and recruiting them into the project. This type of field-work has a long tradition among drug abuse researchers in the United States, and in the majority of cases former drug users or others who have contacts in and/or credibility with networks of drug users are employed to do the job. In Rio de Janeiro, however, there is much less of a tradition, if any at all. After a variety of different recruitment tactics were tried, the project shifted from the idea of a traditional outreach staff to the exclusive use of client recruiters. With specialized training and focus groups, the client recruiters were able to fulfill all of the project's sampling needs.[2]

The lesson here is that in addition to the obvious cultural differences that must be analyzed and reconciled, there are many more subtle ones that also must be discovered. Many folkways, mores, and practices may be so routine to staff members at the international site that they may not be even thought about until they are violated. Moreover, because of the different levels of experience and alternative approaches to research methods seen in the international sector, all aspects of research implementation require constant monitoring.

Language Differences and Translation Problems

Differences in language between the U.S. investigators and both staff and clientele at the research site result in a significant level of extra work. All forms and questionnaires must be translated and back-translated, manuals and other documents must be prepared in two languages, reports and publications must be written for both English and foreign language journals, presentations may require having an interpreter on hand, and all communication involves one or more parties for whom English (or some other language) is a second language. All of this adds an inordinate amount of time to routine tasks. In fact, because of cultural and language differences, even the more mundane tasks often take at least twice the amount of time they otherwise would. And although an investigator might be highly proficient in the language of the international site, or vice versa, there are so many different language nuances and idioms that disasters can and do necessarily occur.

In this HIV/AIDS research endeavor, the coprincipal investigator based in the United States had significant fluency in Brazilian Portuguese. In Brazil, the project's executive director had excellent English skills, and two others had a good understanding of English. No others were bilingual. There were many minor translation errors that occurred almost daily, and one major mistranslation that had a significant financial implication for the project.

As noted earlier, less than a year into the project, and after more than a decade of devastating inflation, Brazil stabilized its currency. However, because the currency was being artificially stabilized through government supports, the U.S. dollar became extremely weak in Brazil. And because salaries were based on the dollar, all staff members experienced the equivalent of a 20 percent pay cut. To compensate, the principal investigator authorized a "one-time only bonus of 16 percent," to be added to the next month's pay check, and only to the next pay check. Although it was explained that the 16 percent bonus was a fringe benefit that should occur only on one pay check, it was interpreted to mean "a 16 percent pay increase" for every staff member. Not surprisingly, the error had some budgetary implications.

Staff Training

A number of decisions about training procedures must be made during the grant-writing phase. Is it more cost-effective to bring key staff members to the United States for training, or is it better to send the trainers to the research site? There is no clear answer for this, because there are likely good reasons to do either or both, depending on the nature of the research and setting. For this Brazil-based research, a similar project was occurring at the University of Miami, and as such, it offered key Brazilian staff the opportunity to have hands-on training in a similar, "live" project. Although this served to be an excellent training experience, it was also quite expensive. Miami researchers also traveled to Brazil to conduct training seminars. On the whole, because of the need for refresher training seminars, new instruments and techniques, and staff turnover, the great majority of the training was done in Brazil by the principal and co-principal investigators.

Researchers must also anticipate that in addition to language differences, cultural differences will increase training time and effort. For example, midway into the project a trailer instrument was added to the cadre of questionnaires, designed to elicit information about (among other things) children in the client's household. One of the questions read as follows:

> I have a few questions about who lives with you. When I ask about children, I mean biological, adopted, step-children, or other children who live in the same house with you. How many children:
>
> A. 2 years or younger are living in the same house with you?
> B. 3–5 years are living in the same house with you?
> C. 6–17 years are living in the same house with you?
> D. 18 years or older are living in the same house with you?

This seemingly straightforward query instigated a two-hour discussion as to what constituted a "child" in one's household. One of the many difficulties with the question in the Brazilian context, for example, was that in many *favela* dwellings there may be several disconnected families living together. As such, whose children are to be considered?

Follow-Up Procedures and Problems

As noted earlier in this chapter, this prevention/intervention project involved a number of steps: (1) client recruitment, (2) intake at the project assessment center (which included informed consent, drug testing, administration the RBA instrument and locator form, and a recruitment trailer form), (3) urine testing, (4) pretest HIV prevention counseling and HIV testing, (5) posttest counseling and furnishing of test results one to three weeks later, and (6) follow-up and reassessment (including HIV testing and counseling) three months later. And because the effectiveness of a project must be determined through follow-up data, it was important that follow-up procedures be well informed before the research begins.

Good follow-up is a combination of art, science, the use of a comprehensive locator form, and a lot of hard work. In Rio de Janeiro, however, the usual techniques for locating clients could not be utilized. Most of the project clients came from the *favelas,* and while these dilapidated shantytowns have many footpaths, trails, passageways, and alleys, there are no formal streets or street names, no addresses, and hence, no mail service. Moreover, there are no telephones. As such, contacting someone to remind them of a follow-up appointment was quite difficult.

Two procedures were put into place to ensure an acceptable level of client retention. First, all clients were given a stipend or R$10 (equivalent to about US$10) for each and every contact at the project office (initial assessment, posttest, and all follow-up contacts). Since the monthly minimum wage was about R$100 during the second and third years of the project, this stipend was considered by most of the clients to be a reasonably good amount of money. Second, the client recruiters were given a bounty of R$10 for each client they physically located and brought to the project office—not only at initial assessment, but at follow-up as well. In addition, client recruiters were given travel coupons for public transportation, which they passed on to clients as an additional inducement to appear.

These procedures yielded retention rates high enough to provide significant numbers of cases to analyze behavioral changes from initial assessment to follow-up. Although these approaches may be useful in other developing communities where slums and shantytowns predominate, investigators considering follow-up studies in international settings must intensively explore the physical and social ecology of their intended target areas to determine appropriate fieldwork strategies.

Postscript

The Rio-based HIV prevention/intervention project had a history longer than most research endeavors. Based on information collected during several trips to Brazil during 1989 through 1991, combined with extensive literature and data searches during the same period, the grant application for the project was written during the closing months of 1991, and submitted to the Division of Research Grants at the National Institutes of Health on January 2, 1992. When it was reviewed during March 1992 it received a priority score of 115, placing close to the top of NIDA's funding list. During the United States–Brasil Binational Research Meeting on Drug Abuse Research in São Paulo on May 21–23, 1992 (see Monteiro and Inciardi 1993), a representative from the National Institute on Drug Abuse proudly announced that his agency's first Brazil-based research project would be funded the following month, with fieldwork scheduled to begin by September, 1992. The principal investigator shared his optimism, but it quickly became apparent that an on-time start-up was not meant to be. As discussed earlier, there were the OPRR project assurances that had to be established and guaranteed, and there were the many clearances from the profusion of U.S. and Brazilian agencies. Rather than June 1992, funding did not occur until some 14 months later. The projected start date for fieldwork was also an illusion. Rather than taking three months to equip a site and hire and train personnel, the complexities associated with these tasks caused the overall process to meander on for more than twice the anticipated time.

An additional point to be emphasized here is that because of the numerous cultural, linguistic, administrative, and bureaucratic differences evident in many developing nations, tasks that may be easy and routine in the United States can be quite complex elsewhere. In Rio de Janeiro, for example, such things as having an office telephone line installed, obtaining someone to fix office plumbing problems, or negotiating the movement of a case of condoms through customs can be major, enduring, and time-consuming operations. Moreover, on-site monitoring of research operations can be very labor intensive. Although the principal investigator had anticipated his travel to Brazil to be only twice annually, the number of necessary site visits turned out to be five to six each year, with a minimum of two researchers traveling to Rio de Janeiro on each occasion.

Yet despite the scores of difficulties, disruptions, and delays, the project accomplished what it had set out to do (see Chapter 4). By the end of its second year of operation, a representative of the Brazilian Ministry of Health informally reported that the project was the largest HIV/AIDS prevention/intervention initiative for drug users in all of Brazil, and that it was being adopted as a national model for reducing AIDS risks among cocaine injectors and snorters.

Notes

1. The NIDA "Standard Intervention" has been reproduced in Appendix A of this book. A copy of this intervention in Brazilian Portuguese can be obtained at

no cost by writing to James A. Inciardi, Center for Drug and Alcohol Studies, University of Delaware, 77 East Main Street, Newark, DE 19716.

2. The "client recruiter" training included some of the basic principles of outreach, and tutoring in the project's protocols, purposes, and human subjects' protections. The recruiters were provided with project tee-shirts and temporary identification cards, and because they were representing the project, they had to abide by a number of rules. Specifically, they could not use drugs or engage in sex with project clients; use drugs, talk about drugs, or be "high" on project property; bring clients who were high; participate in urine exchanges with clients prior to drug testing; ask clients their HIV status. Finally, the recruiters were required to follow a schedule as to when they could bring in new clients.

4

HIV/AIDS Prevention–Intervention in Rio de Janeiro

With the onset of the 1990s, researchers and scientists began reporting that indigent populations were becoming increasingly vulnerable to infection with HIV/AIDS (Walton 1990; Krueger et al. 1990). As the epidemic continues to evolve, global patterns of HIV infection support this premise. Africa, for example, contains 26 of the world's poorest 35 countries, and as noted in the opening chapter of this book, is estimated to have the highest number of HIV-infected people in the world (UNAIDS 1998). These high rates of infection are inextricably linked to conditions of underdevelopment (Ankrah 1991). Even in developed nations, socially marginalized groups including ethnic minorities, low-income persons, and women are now disproportionately represented among HIV/AIDS cases (Montoya et al. 1997; UNAIDS 1998). Studies linking HIV and socioeconomic status have indicated that the pattern of higher infection rates among ethnic minorities corresponds to the proportions of blacks, Hispanics, and whites living below the poverty line (Males 1996). Among women, economic linkages to HIV infection may be even more pronounced because sex- and drug-related transmission are tethered to the social and economic relations of race, class, and gender (Zierler and Krieger 1997).

Brazil evidences many of the conditions of poverty in which HIV/AIDS seems to flourish. Although in the early days of the epidemic AIDS was incorrectly viewed by the Brazilian public as a disease solely affecting wealthy gay men, it was indeed the case that most of those first infected had at least a secondary school education (UNAIDS 1998; Brazilian Ministry of Health 1998). However, the social and economic profile of the epidemic has changed dramatically, and overall the disease is moving into younger, more impoverished and more rural populations (Brazilian Ministry of Health 1998; Daniel and Parker 1993). Because Brazil uses education as an indicator of socioeconomic status, it is significant that as of 1997 more than 60 percent of all registered AIDS cases had occurred among those with only primary school education (UNAIDS 1998; Brazilian Ministry of Health 1998). Although men who have sex with men comprise a large proportion of the population with AIDS, cases acquired through injection drug use or heterosexual transmission have shown the largest increases since the beginning of the AIDS epidemic in Brazil almost two decades years ago.

Although injection drug use is a primary vector of HIV transmission in Brazil, there are few published studies describing the epidemiology of HIV infection in chronic drug using populations. Studies of noninjecting drug users and drug-related sexual risk behaviors are similarly limited. While some small-scale studies have been conducted, the general focus has been on in-treatment populations, oftentimes to the exclusion of street-based users. Because drug treatment programs in Brazil are restricted almost entirely to religious institutions and expensive private clinics (Barbosa de Carvalho et al. 1996), indigent drug users have often been ignored and are virtually unstudied.

The paucity of attention to economically deprived injecting and noninjecting drug users in Brazil demonstrates that, until recently, they were not targeted by HIV prevention initiatives and reflects the widespread social marginalization of the drug-using population. Within this context, this chapter examines the nature of the HIV/AIDS epidemic among marginalized drug users in Rio de Janeiro, with a specific focus on the structure and effectiveness of the HIV prevention program implemented by the authors.

Favela and *Asfalto*

Project recruitment was conducted in a variety of target areas by outreach workers who were indigenous to the areas in which they were recruiting research participants. Rather that full-time outreach workers, however, the project used "client recruiters" to fulfill this function. That is, and as described in detail in Chapter 3, the project relied on its own clients to recruit other clients (Inciardi and Surratt 1997).

The majority of the clients came from several of Rio de Janeiro's many *favelas*. Clustered on the hills and mountainsides that overlook Rio's fashionable beaches and elegant shopping and high-rise centers, the *favelas* are slums in which only a small portion of households have electricity, running water, or sewage facilities. Juramento, for example, like most other *favelas*, is a self-contained realm of the very poor, with 30,000 residences and a dozen or so entry points (Rambali 1993). There is no glass in the windows of the shacks, no electricity or water other than what can be tapped from city lines, and when it rains the gutters run with mud and refuse. The hill is riddled with alleys and passageways, but there are no official street names, and no mail service or telephone lines (Guillermo-prieto 1990).

The appearance and multiplication of the *favelas* in Rio de Janeiro was generally linked to increased poverty, in both relative and absolute terms. The inability of the government to allot sufficient resources to the low-income housing sector resulted in the confinement of the poor to territories devoid of basic infrastructure—most often on unoccupied government lands located under overpasses, marsh areas, or on the slopes of hills (Scholl 1997). *Favelas* are extraterritorial zones controlled by drug traffickers, where the absence of the public authorities (federal, state, or municipal) is almost complete. Just the minimum services required to ensure the survival of the population are provided. Although the government does finance day-care centers, schools, and medical stations, salaries are minimal and usually late, and the quality of teaching and caretaking is low. In addition, the lack of medicines and the reduced number of physicians providing services in these areas present further problems. The unhealthy environment obviously impacts the residents' health, but lacking resources they often resort to *curandeiros* (witch doctors), *rezadeiras* (medicine women), and self-medication (Scholl 1997).

It is estimated that over one million people are currently living in Rio de Janeiro's more than 545 *favelas.* The high population density in the *favelas* has led residents to build shacks with multiple floors, and oftentimes attachments are built onto existing structures to house new arrivals. Space is limited to such a degree that as one resident put it, "Here, when you are cutting onions the neighbor downstairs cries." Another woman spoke about being powerless to prevent more people from moving to her community and building more shacks on the few remaining lots:

When the drug dealers issue an order there's no saying no. Just the other day, a guy pulled a 38 caliber piece and told me: Ma'am, you are complicating things. If you go on trying to bust my plans I'm going to call the guys and ask them to blow out your brains. What was I supposed to do? I just let him be and build his shack.

The balance of the clients were recruited from the *asfalto,* or asphalt sections of the city. The term asphalt refers to districts of the city that contain at least basic infrastructure, such as the Copacabana and Lapa sections of Rio de Janeiro (described in detail in Chapter 6).

Contacts were made on the street and in the *favelas* using standard multiple-starting-point snowball sampling techniques (Inciardi 1986).

Study participants were recruited from low-income neighborhoods and "red light" districts of Rio de Janeiro where rates of drug use and drug selling are high, and from several of Rio de Janeiro's *favelas* including Mangueira, Telégrafo, and Parque Candelária. These are typical *favelas* located in close proximity to the project's assessment center. Because *favelas* are generally closed communities that are hostile to outsiders, access to the *favelas* was obtained through informal agreements made between project staff and *favela* community leaders. And although the client recruiters/outreach workers were residents of the *favela* or downtown neighborhoods where they worked, only those who had access to and credibility with local drug user networks were used.

All contacts in the street and in the *favelas* represented screening interviews. During or after each screening interview, at a time when the rapport between recruiter and respondent was felt to be at its highest level, each respondent was asked to identify other drug users with whom he or she was acquainted. These individuals, in turn, were located and interviewed, and the process was repeated until the social network surrounding each user was exhausted. Although the plan did not ensure a totally unbiased sample, the use of multiple "starting points" eliminated the problem of drawing all respondents from only one social network.

Client recruiters engaged potential respondents in a preliminary discussion of AIDS prevention. These screening interviews included discussions of the project's requirements, including interviews, voluntary HIV testing, and pretest and posttest counseling sessions. A transportation stipend was provided for all client trips. Recruiters also received payment for each client brought to the project center for both initial and follow-up sessions, thereby helping increase follow-up data collection. Eligible participants had to be at least 18 years of age, not in drug treatment or jail during the month prior to interview, and to have reported cocaine use during the thirty days prior to interview.

Prevention–Intervention

The intervention used in the Rio de Janeiro project was grounded in the Health Belief Model, which "attempts to explain and predict health behaviors by focusing on the attitudes and beliefs in individuals" (AIDSCAP 1996). The Health Belief Model, which holds that in order to effect changes in behavior, individuals must (1) attain a certain level of relevant health knowledge, (2) perceive their own vulnerability to a serious health risk, (3) be convinced that changing their behavior will be beneficial in terms of reducing their susceptibility to the health risk, and (4) believe that the benefits of taking action outweigh any risks or drawbacks (Rosenstock et al. 1994). The Health Belief Model has been shown to be a useful framework for examining the impact of other AIDS prevention projects sponsored and funded by the National Institute on Drug Abuse (McBride et al. 1998).

The use of the Health Belief Model as "an active behavior change strategy" (versus a predictive one) in the Rio-based project was a unique use of the model (Inciardi and Surratt 2000). Project educational objectives included client recognition of

1. the severity of AIDS,
2. behaviors that make clients susceptible to contracting HIV,
3. barriers that can block the adoption of risk reduction behaviors,
4. benefits of specific HIV risk reduction behaviors, and
5. the knowledge that drug users have the capability (self-efficacy) to use risk reduction methods.

Overall, the project followed the NIDA protocols noted in Chapter 3 with few adjustments. Slight modifications included a focus on cocaine users (mostly snorters) due to the virtual absence of other drug use (except for marijuana) in Rio de Janeiro. In addition, the project used a "first generation" intervention rather than expanding the NIDA protocols to include any form of enhanced intervention. The "first generation" approach was chosen as a result of input from Brazilian scientists and local health education professionals. HIV prevention research was in its early stages in Brazil when the project began, and it was anticipated that complex random assignments into alternative intervention groups might not be manageable. Therefore, the choice was made to implement only a basic pre-/post-intervention design.

All interviewing, testing, and counseling procedures were conducted at the project assessment center located at the State University of Rio de Janeiro. The baseline contact consisted of the following (Inciardi and Surratt 2000; Inciardi et al. 1997):

1. Screening for drug use by urinalysis to establish eligibility for project involvement, explanation of project goals and purposes, reading and discussion of the consent forms, and signing of form by consenting individuals.
2. Oral administration of RBA questionnaire by a project interviewer. A variety of areas were covered including demographic and socioeconomic information, sexual risk behavior, drug use within the last 30 days, drug treatment history, health status, HIV status, belief of risk for HIV, and arrest history. The RBA discussed the above areas at length, affording participants the opportunity to consider their drug use and sex practices within the context of risky behaviors.

3. Pretest HIV counseling (including HIV risk reduction intervention) and blood testing. Pretest HIV counseling was conducted by counselors specifically trained in HIV issues. Counseling involved an explanation of the voluntary nature of the testing as well as the testing process and potential results. Other topics included HIV disease, transmission routes, risky behaviors, risks associated with cocaine use, demonstration/rehearsal of condom use, stopping unsafe sex practices, communication with sexual partners, cleaning and disinfection of injection equipment, demonstration/rehearsal of needle and syringe cleaning, disposal of hazardous waste material, stopping unsafe drug use, benefits of drug treatment, and mechanisms for reducing risk (Inciardi and Surratt 2000). Participants who chose to do so were then tested by a phlebotomist,[1] and the counselor scheduled a posttest counseling session (approximately two to three weeks from the time of testing).
4. Distribution of cash travel stipend and hygiene kit. All participants, regardless of willingness to undergo HIV testing, were given a cash travel stipend and hygiene kit. The hygiene kit contained AIDS prevention brochures, male and female condoms, bleach, alcohol swabs, and local drug treatment service information.

Posttest counseling involved the reporting and discussion of HIV test results, reinforcement of prevention messages, and advice on practicing healthy behaviors. For most participants, posttest counseling occurred approximately three weeks after intake. The posttest counseling session also served as a booster HIV risk-reduction session, following the format of that used during intake. Participants were encouraged to share their HIV status with any sex and/or drug injection partners. Those who tested positive for HIV were referred to the University hospital for further treatment and counseling.[2]

An effort was made to reassess all participants at a follow-up session three to five months later, with a standardized Risk Behavior Follow-Up Assessment (RBFA) interview instrument and urine testing for cocaine use, followed by HIV retesting and counseling for previously seronegative clients.

Research Findings

Between March 1994 and October 1997, a total of 1,544 cocaine users were recruited, interviewed, and provided the HIV/AIDS intervention program. Because the *favela* and *asfalto* samples appeared to be different on many of the demographic and behavioral dimensions examined, the data for each group are presented separately. As illustrated in Table 4.1, the respondents in both samples were young, with median ages of 28 years for the *favela* residents and 30 years for the *asfalto*. Overall, 22.5 percent of the sample was female, however, significantly more women were recruited from the *favelas* (27.0%) than from the asphalt (16.8%), p<.01. The three predominate race/ethnic categories in Rio de Janeiro—white, black (Afro-Brazilian), and multiracial—were well represented in the total sample, although whites comprised a significantly larger proportion of the asphalt sample (36.9%) than the *favela* (22.6%), p<.01 . The overwhelming majority of participants had minimal education, however, the *favela* residents were particularly disadvantaged, with only 3.4 percent completing high school (p<.01). Income is another indicator of socioeconomic status that finds members of the *favela* sample to be disproportionately represented in the lowest wage categories. The income of the *asfalto* sample was by no means high, however. In fact, for both groups the median income fell between $100 and $300 per month, although the *asfalto* members had a significantly higher mean monthly income (p<.01).

In terms of drug use, both samples were similar in patterns of onset and current use. The data in Table 4.2 indicate that most of the respondents began using alcohol, marijuana, and cocaine in their middle teenage years. Alcohol use in the 30 days prior to interview was reported by 89.7 percent of the *favela* sample, and 90.7 percent of the *asfalto* sample. Marijuana use was less prevalent in both samples—56.3 percent of the *favela* sample and 61.9 percent of the *asfalto* sample reported any use in the past thirty days. As would be expected given the eligibility criteria for the study, 100 percent of the sample reported cocaine use in this 30-day period. Inhalant use was infrequent, with only 2.2 percent of the total sample reporting any lifetime use. Other drugs, such as heroin, crack cocaine, amphetamines, and hallucinogens are not listed because they are generally unavailable in Rio de Janeiro. During the 30-day period prior to being enlisted into the project, alcohol and marijuana use was reported on a median of 12 days, while cocaine use was reported on 16 days. On average, respondents in both samples had been cocaine involved for 11 years. Sample differences emerged in two areas related to drug use. First, *favela* residents were less likely than *asfalto* residents to report ever injecting drugs (12.2% vs. 26.7%), p<.01, and were less likely to have received any type of treatment for substance abuse (4.2% vs. 12.5%), p<.01.

In addition to drug-related behaviors, sexual risks among the participants were not uncommon. As illustrated in Table 4.3, slightly more than one-fourth had multiple sex partners in the month prior to interview. Participation in sex for money exchanges occurred among approximately

TABLE 4.1   Demographic Characteristics of 1,544 Cocaine Users in
Rio de Janeiro, Brazil, 1998

	Favela N=855	Asfalto N=689	Total N=1,544
Age at Interview			
18–24	32.6%	24.7%	29.1%
25–34	39.3%	45.4%	42.0%
35+	28.1%	29.9%	28.9%
Median	28.0%	30.0%	29.0%
*Gender**			
Male	73.0%	83.2%	77.5%
Female	27.0%	16.8%	22.5%
*Ethnicity**			
Black	37.8%	29.6%	34.1%
White	22.6%	36.9%	29.0%
Multiracial	39.6%	33.2%	36.8%
Education			
Less than 12 Years	96.6%	83.9%	90.9%
More than 12 Years	3.4%	16.1%	9.1%
*Monthly Income**			
Less than $100	38.6%	34.7%	36.9%
$101–$300	46.6%	45.2%	45.9%
$301+	14.7%	20.0%	17.1%

*Samples statistically different at p<.01

21 percent of the participants. Significant proportions of both samples also reported histories of sexually transmitted diseases, although rates of STDs were higher among *asfalto* residents (46.7%) than *favela* residents (37.1%), p<.01. This is surprising, given that the rate of condom use among clients from the *asfalto* was significantly higher than among the *favela* residents (p<.01). The rate of HIV infection was also significantly higher among the *asfalto* residents (11.3% vs. 6.5%), p<.01.

Of the 1,544 cocaine users recruited into the prevention/intervention program, 8.7 percent tested positive for antibodies to HIV. As indicated in Table 4.4, multivariate logistic regression analyses found that the risk factors significantly related to HIV seropositivity included having ever injected drugs (p=.003), having traded sex for money (p<.001), having a history of infection with one or more STDs (p=.003), and living in the *asfalto* areas of the city (p=.025). Surprisingly, none of the other variables in

TABLE 4.2   Drug Use Histories of 1,544 Cocaine Users in
Rio de Janeiro, Brazil, 1998

	Favela N=855	Asfalto N=689	Total N=1,544
Median Age at First Use			
Alcohol	15.0	15.0	15.0
Marijuana	16.0	16.0	16.0
Cocaine	16.0	17.0	17.0
Median Days Using in Last 30 Days			
Alcohol	12.0	12.0	12.0
Marijuana	12.0	12.0	12.0
Cocaine	16.0	16.0	16.0
Percent Ever Injecting Drugs*	12.2%	26.7%	18.7%
Ever in Drug Treatment*	4.2%	12.5%	7.9%

*Samples statistically different at p<.01

TABLE 4.3   Sexual Risk Behaviors and HIV Status of 1,544 Cocaine Users in
Rio de Janeiro, Brazil, 1998

	Favela N=855	Asfalto N=689	Total N=1,544
Number of Sex Partners in Last 30 Days			
0	21.5%	20.4%	21.0%
1	52.9%	51.8%	52.6%
2 or more	25.6%	27.8%	26.4%
Percent with STD History*	37.1%	46.7%	41.5%
Percent Using Condoms*	10.6%	16.1%	13.1%
Percent Trading Sex for Money	19.6%	23.4%	21.3%
Percent HIV+*	6.5%	11.3%	8.7%

*Samples statistically different at p<.01

the model, including condom use, appeared to relate to serostatus. And in particular, because of the elusive concept of race in Brazil, serostatus was unrelated to race/ethnicity.[3]

An attempt was made to recontact the 1,544 participants at three months after the baseline interview. Because traditional follow-up techniques were inappropriate for a population that is virtually without telephones, addresses, and mail service, only 782 of the original 1,544 participants (51%) were relocated and reinterviewed at three months postintervention. Only five *new* cases of HIV infection were detected among previously seronegative clients at follow-up, and as such, seroincidence was not a focus of the outcome analysis. Follow-up data suggested that the intervention was effective at reducing risk for HIV. Significantly fewer days of cocaine use were reported at the three-month interview. Specifically, cocaine use fell from 17.28 days to 12.89 days (p<.000) in the previous 30 days. Additionally, 78 clients (10.0%) had abstained from any cocaine use in the 30 days prior to reassessment. Condom use during vaginal sex increased from a mean of 1.69 times (during the past 30 days) at baseline to 3.71 times at follow-up (p=.003). These changes were not specific to either the *favela* or the *asfalto* group. In other words, both groups appeared to respond equally well to the intervention. Importantly, the follow-up sample was very similar to the baseline sample on a variety of demographic and drug use measures, suggesting that positive outcomes were not attributable to between-group differences resulting from attrition.

The Changing Epidemiology of HIV/AIDS in Brazil

The movement of HIV infection into younger, more impoverished, and more rural populations in Brazil is occurring concurrently with the rise in injection drug-related and heterosexually acquired cases of AIDS. Consequently, as the epidemiology of HIV infection changes, increasing numbers of people who were not targets of early information and prevention campaigns are at significant risk of infection. This project provided an opportunity to penetrate acutely impoverished communities in order to assess HIV risk among previously unstudied cohorts of cocaine users.

The overall rate of HIV infection for this sample was 8.7 percent. This is extremely high, considering that more than 80 percent of the participants had no history of injection drug use. The results of this research are consistent with any number of studies that have found HIV seropositivity to be related to injection drug use, trading sex for money, and having one or more sexually transmitted diseases. One of the most interesting findings was the significantly higher HIV infection rate among the *asfalto* residents

TABLE 4.4   Significant Predictors of HIV Infection for 1,544 Cocaine Users, Rio de Janeiro, Brazil, 1998

	Regression Coefficient	*Odds Ratio*	*95% C.I.*
Asfalto Residence*	.4251	1.530	(1.06, 2.22)
STD History*	.5583	1.748	(1.21, 2.53)
Drug Injection History*	.6163	1.852	(1.24, 2.77)
Sex Trading History*	.7841	2.190	(1.49, 3.22)

*Reference category is "no." Nonsignificant predictors included age, race/ethnicity, gender, level of education, income, length of cocaine use, drug treatment history, number of sexual partners in the past 30 days, and condom use in the past 30 days.

than that of the *favela* residents (11.3% vs. 6.5%). This relationship is maintained even when participants with a history of injection drug use are excluded from the analysis. That is, cocaine snorters from the *asfalto* areas of the city remained significantly more likely to be HIV-positive than cocaine snorters from *favela* communities (9.3% vs. 5.7%, p=.01).

Participants from both the *asfalto* and the *favela* communities displayed high levels of HIV risk behaviors. However, there were key differences in their injection drug use, condom use, and histories of sexually transmitted diseases. For example, injection drug use tends to be more common in the *asfalto* areas of Rio de Janeiro because of the higher quality of cocaine available there. In the *favelas,* the cocaine is often "cut" by dealers with any number of substances (i.e., corn flour, fruit salt, sodium bicarbonate, and marble powder), so much so that one kilo is typically expanded to five kilos (Telles et al. 1997; Scholl 1997). A number of these mixtures make injecting difficult, if not impossible. Residents of the *asfalto* were able to purchase cocaine of higher purity suitable for injecting. In addition, they had greater access to needles and syringes sold in pharmacies at relatively low cost.

The extent of participants' condom use was not related to rates of HIV infection, but this may have been due to the nature of the data collection instrument, in that the data on condom usage covered only the 30-day period prior to interview. At the same time, the higher level of condom use among the *asfalto* residents may reflect greater awareness of risk for HIV and other STDs and better access to information on safe sex. Interestingly, however, in contrast to those in the *favelas,* more of the *asfalto* residents had histories of diagnosed STDs, more had been tested previously for HIV, and more had previously received AIDS risk reduction information and supplies. In fact, 10 percent of *asfalto* residents received condoms in the past 30 days compared to 5.3 percent of *favela* residents. These factors are likely a reflection the paucity of medical, health, and social services available in the *favela* communities. In fact, at one point early in the project, the authors visited the medical clinic in Mangueira, a *favela* located not too far from the project headquarters. The available supplies at the clinic included little more than a few packages of basic first aid materials.

Limitations

Despite the compelling nature of the study findings, there were a number of limitations. First, the sampling was not a random design, but this occurred for a number of reasons. Rio de Janeiro is a city with more than 545 *favelas*, yet the project recruited from only a dozen of these communities. Although the *favelas* throughout Rio de Janeiro share certain demographic and economic characteristics, each is controlled by highly territorial drug traffickers, such that residents of one *favela* may be unwelcome and unsafe in another such community. Therefore, sampling was restricted to *favelas* where our outreach workers were known, and it was neither financially nor logistically feasible to retain indigenous outreach workers from hundreds of different *favelas* in order to gain access to these communities. At the same time, recruitment from the *asfalto* sections of the city was also localized, because drug users were concentrated in certain areas and were not randomly distributed. Overall, this tempered our ability to generalize the findings of this study to all of the communities within metropolitan Rio de Janeiro.

A second limitation was related to the use of the standardized RBA instrument. Because the project was one of NIDA's Cooperative Agreement sites (see Chapter 3), a number of procedures were standardized across sites, including much of the instrumentation. Unfortunately, the RBA instrument captured minimal information on *lifetime* HIV sexual risk behaviors and focused heavily on risk behaviors occurring in the past 30 days. This fact limited our ability to document relationships between HIV status, condom use, and number of sexual partners that may have been apparent if historical information were available.

Finally, the preliminary outcome data presented showed the intervention to be successful in decreasing cocaine use while increasing condom use. However, because of the single-group/before-after design, it is impossible to conclude that the intervention caused the positive changes in HIV risk behaviors. In addition, attrition from baseline to follow-up was significant. Those who returned for the follow-up may have been those most motivated to change. However, the positive changes in drug use were unique to cocaine, the only drug specifically targeted by the intervention. There were no changes in either alcohol or marijuana use, suggesting that the intervention had a beneficial impact.

Postscript

Despite these limitations, this study demonstrated the feasibility of accessing impoverished communities using indigenous client recruiters and documented the residents' willingness to participate in an AIDS education/prevention program. Outcome data further suggest that the participants were able to learn and apply specific HIV risk reduction techniques to their behavior in the short term. These findings are particularly important when examined in conjunction with the rate of HIV infection in this population. Although 6.5 percent of the drug users from *favela* communities tested HIV-positive, and 11.3 percent of those from other low-income *asfalto* neighborhoods did so, these rates of infection are significantly *lower* than those documented in populations of lower-middle income drug injectors recruited from treatment programs in Rio de Janeiro (Telles et al. 1997). We believe that the lower HIV prevalence in the most impoverished communities in Rio de Janeiro is primarily a function of two factors. The first is that the initial introduction of HIV to Brazil occurred primarily in the upper and middle classes, beginning with gay and bisexual men, and then drug injectors (Telles et al. 1997). The second factor related to lower HIV infection is the relative social isolation of the *favela* communities. Although the *favelas* are geographically interspersed with the *asfalto* areas of the city, the social distance between the communities is enormous. Many of the *favelas* are mazelike in design and have very few access points that connect to the *asfalto* areas outside. Access to the *favelas* by outsiders, including the police, is extremely limited and, in fact, many residents of the *favelas* do not consider themselves to be citizens of the mainstream or *asfalto* society. Under these conditions, social networks are formed almost exclusively within the *favela,* rather than outside it, and interaction with middle-and upper-society is nonexistent. Because of this pattern of interaction with the larger society, it may be that these impoverished communities have only recently been penetrated by HIV, and therefore are presently evidencing lower rates of infection. As the epidemic continues to unfold and risk among the mass of low-income drug users rises, however, the timely implementation of effective strategies to prevent HIV transmission assumes great importance. The recent opening of a needle/syringe exchange program that serves impoverished drug users in Rio de Janeiro seems to indicate that the community's recognition of an impending crisis is growing. The institutionalization of HIV prevention protocols for drug and sexual risk behaviors into community-based organizations is also desperately needed in order to begin to address the long-term unmet health needs of individuals in these impoverished communities.

Notes

1. HIV testing was done by ELISA, with confirmatory testing through both Western Blot and Indirect Immunofluorescence Assay (IFA) procedures.

2. For a full discussion of the NIDA Standard Intervention and its changes over time, see Wechsberg et al. 1997). A copy of the basics of the intervention appears in Appendix A of this book. A copy in Brazilian Portuguese can be obtained at no charge by writing to James A. Inciardi, Center for Drug and Alcohol Studies, University of Delaware, Newark, DE 19716.

3. For an analysis of the concept of race in Brazil in general, and how it affected the project in particular, see Appendix B.

5

The Female Condom and HIV Risk Reduction

More than one million people in Latin America are currently living with HIV/AIDS, and since the late 1980s this region has experienced dramatic increases in the number of HIV infections acquired through heterosexual contact (WHO 1997; Berkley 1993). Given that male-to-female transmission of HIV is reported to be 24 times more efficient than female-to-male (WHO 1995), the rise in heterosexual transmission has greatly impacted seroprevalence rates among women. Nowhere has this impact been greater than in Brazil, where heterosexual contact is the major mode of transmission for women, and the ratio of male-to-female cases dropped from 25.5:1 in 1985 to 2.1:1 in 1999 (Brazilian Ministry of Health 1999).

Despite the alarming increase in AIDS, the Brazilian government has not focused prevention efforts directly on women. The information, education, and counseling campaigns of Brazil's National Program on STDs/AIDS have generally targeted health professionals and those considered to be engaging in high-risk behaviors: men who have sex with men, injection drug users, commercial sex workers, and adolescents (Center for Reproductive Law and Policy 1995). As a result, many women who do not engage in injection drug use or prostitution do not perceive themselves to be at risk and may do little to change their behaviors (Campbell 1990). Despite the low perception of risk among the general population of women in Brazil, heterosexual contact with a seropositive sex partner continues to present a significant risk for infection. In fact, the greatest need for AIDS education and prevention efforts may be among monogamous married and cohabiting women. For example, a study conducted in São Paulo—Brazil's largest city—found that just under half of all new AIDS cases among women were reported among those who were both married and monogamous (Heise and Elias 1995).

Brazilian cultural norms support notions of male dominance and control in sexual encounters, and as such, many women feel that discussing or negotiating safe sex with their partners is not permissible (Gupta and Weiss 1993). In fact, an extremely large number of Brazilian women have reported choosing sterilization as their method of birth control in order to avoid discussions of contraception with their partners (Gupta and Weiss 1993). For example, the proportion of married women of childbearing age in Brazil reporting the use of condoms was only 2 percent at the close of the 1980s (Goldberg et al. 1989). Similarly, in a study of Brazilian women of childbearing age, it was found that 71 percent used some method of birth control, and of these, 44 percent had been sterilized, 41 percent took oral contraceptives, but less than 2 percent used condoms (Goldstein 1994). In subsequent focus groups with married women, none had broached the subject of condoms with their spouses (Goldstein 1994).

The implications of these data for the spread of HIV among women in Brazil are evident. Although the consistent use of male condoms is demonstrably effective in preventing the spread of HIV, condom use requires a high degree of motivation and cooperation by male partners (Stein 1990, 1995). Oftentimes, women who attempt to negotiate condom use are viewed as unfaithful or too "prepared" for sex (Carovano 1991). These beliefs are most likely a reflection of negative attitudes about condoms in general. Male condoms have long been associated with the prevention of sexually transmitted diseases (STDs) acquired during illicit extramarital relationships (Potts and Short 1989). Other studies have documented equally negative attitudes about condoms, including an adverse effect on sexual enjoyment, discomfort, interference with sex, embarrassment, irritation of the genitalia, less connection to the partner, and perceived lack of trust. Such attitudes are strongly associated with nonuse of condoms (Hetherington et al. 1996; Sacco et al. 1991; Valdiserri et al. 1989).

Research has demonstrated that women have more positive attitudes about condom use than men, but are no more likely to use condoms because of male resistance (Sacco et al. 1991). And until only recently, there were NO woman-controlled methods of sexual risk reduction available to women at risk of HIV infection. This situation changed dramatically with the introduction of the female condom.

The Introduction of the Female Condom in the Americas

The first female condom, made of rubber with a steel coil rim, was introduced during the early decades of the twentieth century (Editorial 1992). However, it was not until the late 1980s that a more acceptable device was developed—the Femidom™ female condom, which has been commercially available in the United Kingdom since September 1992 and received approval from the Food and Drug Administration for distribution in the United States in 1993. Throughout much of the Americas, the female condom is marketed by the Female Health Company under the name of Reality™. As illustrated below, the female condom is a polyurethane sheath with a flexible inner ring, which secures the condom against the cervix, and an outer ring, which prevents the condom from entering the vaginal canal. The design combines features of the male condom and the diaphragm (Bounds et al. 1988).

The female condom has several advantages over the male condom both as a contraceptive and as an STD prevention method. First, it is woman-controlled. With the female condom, women are not as dependent on the cooperation of sex partners to protect themselves from HIV and other sexually transmitted diseases. Second, the female condom is inserted before intercourse, providing additional protection against infections from pre-ejaculated fluids. Third, the female condom protects a greater proportion of the vagina, providing additional protection against STDs. Fourth, the female condom has less risk of rupture than the male condom (Bounds et al. 1988; Bounds 1989; Leeper and Conrardy 1989; Gollub and Stein 1993). Other advantages are that because of its loose fit, it causes less loss of sensitivity, it permits penetration before complete erection of the penis, and it permits continued intimacy in the resolution phase of intercourse since it need not be removed immediately (Bounds et al. 1988).

Various tests have been performed on the female condom with promising results. In a leak test where condoms were tested for pin holes and tears during manufacturing, the female condom received a .6 percent leakage rate compared to a 3.5 percent leakage rate for the male condom. In another leak test measuring spillage during use, the female condom had a 2.7 percent vaginal exposure rating whereas the male condom had a 8.1 percent rating. In 74 episodes in which the female condom was used, there was no incidence of semen in the vagina. The combined risk for the female condom is 3.0 percent and for the male condom it is 11.6 percent (Leeper and Conrardy 1989; Leeper 1990).

In simulated laboratory testing of the female condom, there was no viral leakage for either HIV or cytomegalovirus (Drew et al. 1989). In another viral leakage test, the female condom was found to be highly effective in protecting against exposure to HIV (Voeller 1991). In a quasi-experimental project, 104 women were randomly assigned to an experimental group that used the female condom or to a control group that used no protection. None of the women in the experimental group who previously had vaginal trichomoniasis tested positive for the infec-

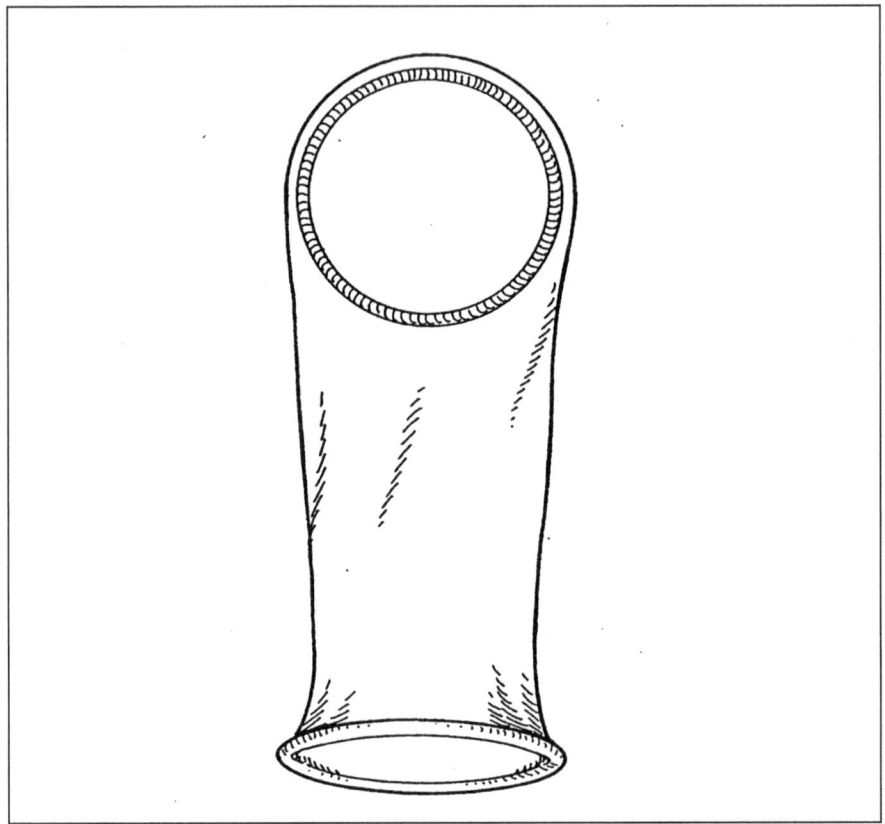

FIGURE 5.1   The Female Condom

tion at follow-up, whereas 14 percent in the control group tested positive for vaginal trichomoniasis (Soper et al. 1993). The female condom has also been found to have no effect on resident bacteria flora and there is no evidence of lower genital tract trauma during intercourse when the female condom is used (Soper et al. 1991).

A number of early studies tested the acceptability of the female condom among both women and men. Of 24 couples studied in the United Kingdom, for example, 67 percent of the women and 83 percent of the men found the female condom easy to use; 50 percent of the women and 54 percent of the men found it an acceptable contraceptive and HIV/STD prevention method; 50 percent of the women and 37 percent of the men preferred it to the male condom (Schilling et al. 1991). In a study of 294 American women, 73 percent found the female condom easy to use, 56 percent considered it an acceptable contraceptive, and 82 percent found it

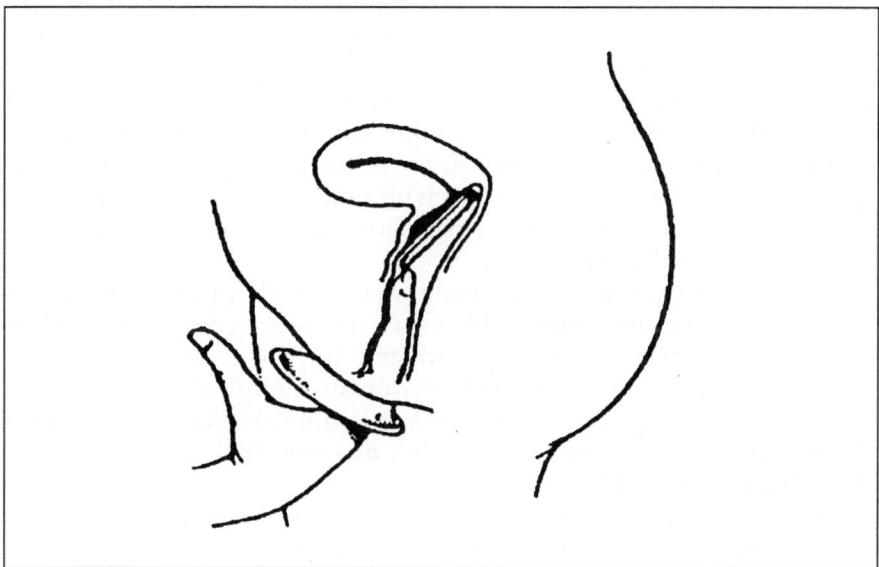

FIGURE 5.2   Female Condom Insertion

an acceptable HIV/STD prevention method (Schilling et al. 1991). Another early U.S. study examined the attitudes toward and acceptance of the female condom among minority women. The sample included 20 African-American and 37 Latina women in a methadone maintenance program. The respondents did not use the condom but were interviewed on their acceptance of it after being educated about it. More than 75 percent of the women had favorable attitudes toward the female condom, 63 percent of their steady partners had favorable attitudes, and 65 percent of the women thought the female condom would be easier to use than the male condom (Schilling et al. 1991).

Prior to the introduction of the female condom in the United States, few studies of the acceptability of the female condom had been conducted among women at high risk for HIV, and in most, samples had been extremely small. In Thailand, for example, 20 sex workers were educated about and given female condoms. The female condom was used in 32 percent of all sexual encounters and male condoms in 35 percent. Almost all the women—90 percent—said they would recommend the female condom to friends (Sakondhavat 1990). Twenty-four prostitutes in Mexico had also been educated about the female condom. Twenty-one agreed to use it and 18 were interviewed at a later date about acceptance and use. After becoming accustomed to using the female condom, respondents found it to be more protective against HIV and STD infection.

The respondents also found female condoms more feasible to use than male condoms in that the former were more adaptable to their lifestyle. For example, respondents successfully learned to hide the outer ring of the female condom from clients to avoid discussion of condom use. (This was accomplished by pushing the outer ring into the vagina and then pulling it back out immediately prior to intercourse.) Many of the respondents used the female condom with regular sex partners, and both the respondents and their regular partners found the female condom acceptable (Hernandez-Avila 1992).

The major advantage of the female condom is that women are not as dependent on the cooperation of their sex partners to protect themselves from HIV and other STDs (Gollub and Stein 1993; Shervington 1993). The female condom, moreover, is the only woman-controlled device that has been approved by the U.S. Food and Drug Administration specifically for the prevention of sexually transmitted diseases, including HIV/AIDS (Gollub and Stein 1993).

When the female condom first became available in the United States in 1994, the media response was less than enthusiastic. Many articles focused on the reactions of middle-class women who were not at particularly high risk for HIV. The condom was compared to a plastic sock, a vacuum cleaner bag, a parched jellyfish, a "Trojan" on steroids, a "Hefty" bag, an elephant's trunk, and a windsock (Blumenfeld 1992; Jackson 1994). It was also reported to make crude noises, cause a loss of sensation, feel strange, and prevent women from feeling "what's going on" (Jackson 1994).

On the other hand, the initial reactions from women at a significant risk for HIV infection were far more positive. A recent study of 37 injection drug users and crack cocaine users, for example, reported at least one-time use of the female condom by 80 percent of the participants (Ashery et al. 1995). Moreover, in a study of 231 women recruited from STD and public health clinics, those who had no prior knowledge of the condom were more likely to try it than those who had already heard of it (Sly et al. 1997), suggesting that the initial negative commentary may have discouraged some women from using it. Given the traditionally low rates of male condom usage in both general and high-risk populations in the U.S. and abroad (Calsyn et al. 1992; Goldberg et al. 1989), it was important to assess Brazilian women's attitudes and reactions to this new HIV risk reduction device.

The Female Condom in Brazil

During the closing months of 1995, the authors conducted the first public conference forum in Brazil on the use of the female condom (Inciardi and

Surratt 1995). Sample female condoms were provided to the members of the audience, and the response was highly positive. At the time, the female condom was not commercially available, and generally unknown, in Brazil. Several months later, the authors initiated a pilot project in Rio de Janeiro to systematically examine the acceptability of the female condom among drug-involved women. Established with the approval of the Brazilian Ministry of Health (Surratt, et al.1999), the study was conducted in conjunction with the HIV/AIDS prevention effort in Rio de Janeiro described in Chapters 3 and 4.

During the pretest counseling phase of the intervention, both male and female clients were introduced to the female condom. Interventionists discussed the advantages of the female condom, including its importance as a woman-controlled device and its utility in the prevention of HIV and other STDs. Differences between the male and female condom were explained, as were instructions for its proper insertion and use and techniques for negotiating condom use with sex partners. Both male and female clients were included in this phase of the intervention, and all were asked to perform the insertion technique on an anatomically correct vaginal model. In order to reduce the anxiety of some respondents, a pelvic model was used to demonstrate precisely how the female condom fit and conformed to the woman's reproductive tract. The participants practiced the insertion on the model until they were comfortable with the procedure and with handling the condom. At the close of this session, each client received two female condom "starter packs" containing three condoms, a tube of lubricant, literature, and illustrated instructions. Women and men alike were asked to try the female condom with their partners.

During the second intervention session one to three weeks later, respondents were asked about their experiences with the female condom—whether they used it and in what situations, and how they and their sex partners felt about it. In addition, all female respondents were given a booster session on the insertion and use of the female condom, and were asked to participate in the follow-up study (if they intended to be sexually active during the study period). Those who agreed were given an adequate supply of female condoms and were asked to return for a follow-up interview three months later. A brief follow-up instrument focused on such issues as frequency of female condom use, ease/problems of use, likes and dislikes, partner reactions, aesthetic issues, and potential use in the future.

Table 5.1 illustrates the background characteristics of the 122 women who received the female condom intervention and subsequently returned for posttest counseling. Their median age was 28 years, and the majority (52.5%) were single. Participants identified themselves most of-

TABLE 5.1   Selected Demographic Characteristics of 122 Female Respondents

Median Age	28.0
Marital Status	
Single	52.5%
Married/Living with Partner	35.3%
Separated	9.8%
Widowed	2.5%
Race/Ethnicity	
Black	34.4%
White	18.9%
Multiracial	46.7%
Education	
Less than 8 years	93.5%
More than 8 years	6.5%

ten as multiracial (46.7%), followed by black (34.4%), and white (18.9%). Because most of the women were recruited from Rio de Janeiro's *favelas* (79.5%) and other impoverished communities, educational levels were low, with almost 94 percent completing fewer than eight years of school. Furthermore, the majority (51.6%) earned less than one "minimum salary," which was equivalent to about US $100 per month.

As illustrated in Table 5.2, almost a fourth of the respondents mentioned a history of sex trading. In addition, 11.4 percent had multiple sexual partners during the previous 30 days. Moreover, almost all (87.7%) reported no use of male condoms in the 30 days prior to the first interview. Although many of the women were engaging in unprotected sex, nearly two-thirds believed that they had *no* chance of becoming infected with HIV. And in fact, the HIV infection rate was a relatively low 2.5 percent.

When asked at the second interview whether they had used the female condom for vaginal sex, 56.6 percent of the women reported having done so. When examining only those 97 women who reported sexual activity, the percentage who tried the condom increased to 71.1 percent. Multivariate logistic regression analyses were used to investigate the relationship between use of the female condom and its possible correlates. As Table 5.3 illustrates, occasions of vaginal sex, residence in a *favela*, having adult family in the household, and perceived risk for AIDS comprised the model predicting female condom use in the Rio de Janeiro pilot study. Of these factors, however, only "perceived risk for AIDS" was statistically significant (p=.027).

TABLE 5.2   Sexual Behavior, HIV Risk, and Serostatus of 122 Female Respondents

*Number of Sex Partners**

0	23.0%
1	65.6%
2 or more	11.4%

Sex Trading

Percent Yes	24.6%

*Any Male Condom Use**

Percent Yes	12.3%

Perceived AIDS Risk

No Chance	66.4%
Some Chance	33.6%

HIV Status

Negative	97.5%
Positive	2.5%

*Time period referenced is the 30 days prior to interview

TABLE 5.3   Logistic Regression Model of Female Condom Use

	Regression Coefficient	*Odds Ratio*	*95% C.I.*
Occasions of Vaginal Sex	.023	1.024	(.998, 1.049)
Favela Residence[a]	.911	2.487	(.913, 6.773)
Perceived Risk of Living with AIDS[ab]	.993	2.700	(1.115, 6.534)
Living with Adult Family[a]	-.778	.459	(.207, 1.016)

[a]Significant at p=.05.
[b]Reference category is "no."
NOTE: Model chi-square=18.56 (p=.001).

Regardless of their reported use or nonuse of the female condom at the first data collection point, sexually active women who expressed a desire to participate were enrolled into the follow-up study, and 53 women ultimately returned for the three-month follow-up interview. Of these, 33 (62.3%) used the female condom at least once over the three-month period. All of the women using the condom tried it with their main sexual partner (husband or boyfriend) and very few felt that the condom would provoke violent or emotionally abusive reactions in their partners. Of those not using the condom on some occasions, four reported male partners objecting, but otherwise the women indicated that it was *their* choice not to use it.

Examining continued use of the female condom as a measure of acceptability, 23 women (43.4%) reported using it for vaginal sex on four or more occasions. When contrasted against women who tried the female condom only once or not at all, two significant associations were found. Users of male condoms at follow-up were 5.5 times more likely than non-users to adopt the female condom as well (p=.018). By contrast, women living in *favelas* were much less likely to continue using the female condom than were nonresidents (p=.004). No other factors included in the model were found to be associated with continued use of the female condom.

The Female Condom and the Culture of the *Favelas*

Because of problems with attrition in the Rio de Janeiro study combined with its exploratory nature, sample sizes were small at both data collection points. Therefore, the data presented here should not be considered exhaustive. Nevertheless, the findings point to three issues which may help to explain why the female condom received positive responses from some women, and not others, and why many women in the study were quite willing to try this new condom, but not continue using it. The first issue is associated with public perceptions of the female condom, the second involves perceptions of risk for HIV/AIDS, and the third may be directly related to the culture of the Brazilian *favela* (Surratt and Inciardi 1999).

With respect to public perceptions, the introduction of the female condom in the U.S. received considerable attention from the media, much of which focused on negative judgments and opinions of its aesthetic features and the belief that it was yet another device that placed the burden of pregnancy and disease prevention on women (Blumenfeld 1992; Jackson 1994). Because the female condom was not commercially available in Brazil when the authors' pilot project was launched, however, it received almost no publicity. In fact, perhaps the first article to appear in a major Brazilian scientific journal was prepared by the authors of this book. It was a brief column that described the history of the female condom, its initial use in several parts of the world, and its role in STD prevention (Inciardi, et al. 1997). In mid-1997, a second article appeared, reporting on the experiences of 115 middle-class women in a pilot study conducted by the Secretary of Health for the State of São Paulo and Fam-

TABLE 5.4   Logistic Regression Model of *Continued* Female Condom Use

	Regression Coefficient	Odds Ratio	95% C.I.
Favela Residence[a][b]	-2.242	.106	(.02, .48)
Any Male Condom Use[a][b]	1.713	5.55	(1.34, 23.01)

[a]Significant at p=.05.
[b]Reference category is "no."
NOTE: Model chi-square=18.56 (p=.001).

ily Health International (Affonso 1997). That study found that 75 percent of the women liked the female condom. One of the most important reasons cited was that it is woman-controlled, thus making the negotiation of its use easier. The report also indicated that many women from other cities in Brazil had contacted the program because they had learned of its success and were eager to participate. Importantly, negative commentary about the female condom had not appeared in the media prior to the study, and the participants were allowed to draw their own conclusions.

While the research in São Paulo introduced the female condom to a sample of middle-class women, the pilot work described in this chapter targeted indigent women drug users in Rio de Janeiro. As in São Paulo, despite the socioeconomic differences, the levels of acceptance were similar. By contrast, in companion studies with indigent drug-using women in the United States, there was significantly less approval of the female condom (Surratt et al. 1998).

On the issue of risk perceptions, the finding that initial use of the female condom was related to perceived risk for AIDS has an important implication for the design of other prevention/intervention programs. Although there was denial of any AIDS risk by nearly two-thirds of the women studied, those who perceived at least some risk were more likely to use the female condom. This is consistent with other studies that have documented a strong relationship between perceived AIDS risk and changes in sexual behaviors (McBride et al. 1997). Based on these findings, interventions that address denial and attempt to personalize risk for AIDS appear to be warranted.

The three-month follow-up interviews indicated high rates of female condom use for women who returned: 62.3 percent reported trying the condom during at least one occasion of vaginal sex, and 43.4 percent reported continuous use. Although perceived risk for AIDS appeared to influence initial use of the female condom among many women, it did not appear sufficient to sustain this use. Continued use was more likely among users of male condoms. Importantly, however, these women were not users of male condoms at the baseline contact. In other words, it appears that male condom use increased between baseline and follow-up, in conjunction with the use of female condoms. That is, women who adopted one method of risk reduction seemed more likely to use the other as well. This, too, is important for HIV prevention considering that none of the women had ever used female condoms prior to the study and only 12.3 percent had recent experiences with male condoms.

Moving on to the final issue, women living in *favelas* were much less likely to continue using the female condom than were nonresidents, and this is most likely related to the culture of the *favela* and the inferior and subservient roles that women occupy in *favela* life.

Brazil's Municipal Planning Institute has estimated Rio's *favelas* to number 545 at the beginning of the 1990s and to house more than 1 million persons (Loveman 1991), and as noted in earlier chapters, only a small portion of households have electricity, running water, or sewage facilities. In the absence of public medical facilities and unemployment benefits for the many unemployed, disease and social problems are common (Gay 1994; Guillermoprieto 1990).

Fieldwork during the course of the project found that because daily life in the *favelas* is virtually controlled by drug traffickers, the so-called *lei do mais forte* (the law of the strongest) operates. The *chefão* or "big boss" is the man who defeats his enemies by violence. Conflicts are driven by competition for power, for the profits from illegal sales of drugs and weapons, and from kidnappings and robberies. The defeated have their assets and "harem" confiscated. Within this context, women in the *favelas* are seen as objects rather than as actual persons; they are commodities that are fought over, and they are seduced and displayed as trophies (Scholl, 1997).

Among the *favelados*, even if women have some financial autonomy and assume household responsibilities, all decisions are still made by men. Furthermore, women's sexual behavior tends to be strictly and forcefully monitored by family and bystanders alike, but this is rarely the case for men. To avoid being harassed by men, be it bandits or police, poor women choose to find a "protector." In this regard, some women establish relationships with members of the local drug markets. Others may be selected by the traffickers against their will. Whatever the scenario, as wives, girlfriends, or lovers of these men, they acquire a degree of respect from the community.

Such sexual inequality tends to be inversely related to opportunities for sexual decision-making and to socioeconomic status in many parts of the world (Worth 1989; Stein 1990; Gupta and Weiss 1993). This is also the case for Brazilian women living in the *favela*'s culture of poverty. They face a way of life that encompasses sexual domination by men. In fact, it is well known in Brazil that some police officers routinely raid the *favelas*, humiliate its residents, and sexually brutalize a number of its women (Surratt and Inciardi 1999). To some police, poor women are *putas* (whores) who "are there to serve us" (Scholl 1997).

Postscript

It is within the context of these social, cultural, and economic conditions that appropriate HIV/AIDS intervention programs for Brazilian women need to be implemented. Perhaps because the female condom is somewhat of a novelty in Brazil, many women were eager to try it. For the women in Rio de Janeiro's *favela* communities, however, the prospect of permanent adoption of this device as a method of risk reduction remains doubtful. Although the female condom provides some women with another option for disease protection, those women involved in sexually exploitive relationships still do not have the power to exercise protection independently of their partners.

6

Transvestism and HIV/AIDS in Brazil

Cross-dressing, female impersonation, and other types of "gender bending" are commonplace, particularly in the entertainment world where they are designed to confront, shock, and fascinate audiences. For Boy George, David Bowie, Kiss, Mick Jagger, Twisted Sister, and the late Tiny Tim, cross-dressing calls into question the conventional notions of "masculine" and "feminine," "male" and "female," and "man" and "woman." On the stage and in the concert halls, gender bending is generally little more than a confusion of costume; the illusion of assuming the opposite sex is intended to suggest ambiguity, not authenticity. Cross-gender identity, on the other hand, is likely to be a far more common, but infinitely more complex, phenomenon.

Cross-gender identity, the sense of belonging to the gender opposite of one's anatomic sex, has existed throughout history and in all parts of the world despite the clear-cut gender distinctions that most cultures require (Bullough and Bullough 1993). Interestingly, a number of societies also integrate into their clearly defined gender players, a "third" gender role, and thus legitimize the place of ambiguity. For example, Indian society institutionalizes the role of the Hijra who are neither male nor female, but rather, contain elements of both (Nanda 1985). Native American cultures also provide space in the pantheon of gender roles for hermaphrodites.

Cross-Dressing and Transvestism

In Western countries, one of the more popular terms used to designate the range of cross-gender identity is *transvestism* (Latin for "cross-dressing"), coined almost a century ago by the German sexologist, Magnus Hirschfeld (Hirschfeld 1910). Although Hirschfeld identified a variety of different types of transvestites (see Lukianowicz 1959), many of his contemporaries felt that the term was far too literal, and that it overemphasized the importance of clothing and failed to include the "feminine" identity factors present in male cross-dressers.

In contrast, Havelock Ellis (1926) preferred the term *eonism* to transvestism, which he based on a historical personage, the Chevalier d'Eon de Beaumont (1728–1810). At the time of d'Eon's death, an autopsy revealed that he did indeed have the anatomical body parts of a man, yet he lived as a man for only 49 years and as a woman for 34 (Garber 1992). During his lifetime, both the French king and English court had "proved" he was a woman (Garber 1992). The persistence of the Chevalier d'Eon's contemporaries to determine his sex and the consequent ambiguity surrounding the settlement is a telling testimony to society's need to define cross-gender identity. Since that time numerous other terms have been suggested, including "gynemimesis" (literally, "woman mime"), and its counterpart "andromimesis," "gender dysphoria," "female or male impersonation," "transgenderism," "femmiphilia," "androphilia," "femme mimesis," "fetishism," "fetishistic cross-dressing," "crossing," and "transsexualism" (Bullough and Bullough 1993).

Regardless of the many epithets, "transvestism" is the term most commonly seen in both the professional and popular literature. Unfortunately, the word tends to obscure rather than clarify, for it fails to distinguish the motivations, satisfactions, or purposes of cross-dressing. Factoring in the sexual orientation of the cross-dresser only makes the situation even more complex. In Hirschfeld's original conceptualization, transvestism is a sexual variation in itself, and he recognizes that both men and women could be transvestites, and that they could be homosexual, heterosexual, bisexual, or asexual ("automonosexual" in his terms). Some recent analyses, however, suggest that the definition of transvestism requires a heterosexual orientation (Docter 1988:6). To further complicate matters, some in the field of psychiatry accept "transvestism" not only as a term, but also as a diagnosis (Stoller 1971). Finally, several observers argue that since homosexuality (and heterosexuality by implication) is a sexual activity and cross-dressing is primarily a role activity, it is appropriate to refer to homosexuality as a sexual variation and to transvestism as a gender variation (Prince and Bentler 1972).

In Brazil, transvestism is a specific social and cultural construct in which both gender and sexuality are mapped out and performed in highly particular ways (Parker 1989, 1999). Moreover, it has a long history, both as an integral theme during *Carnaval*, and as a gender variation with its own distinct culture (Bloom 1997; Linger 1992; Scheper-Hughes 1992). At *Carnaval*, many males—both gay and heterosexual—participate dressed as women, not only to glorify and venerate women, but also as a projection of male sexual fantasies (Scheper-Hughes 1992). But this recreational cross-dressing is only one-sided; women rarely, if ever, cross-dress in *Carnaval*. The role of women who participate in this festival is to *un*dress, not cross-dress, as the colorful and erotic photos of nude women in the major Brazilian *Carnaval* magazines clearly illustrate (see *Manchete* 1997).

The *Travestis* of Brazil

In contrast to *Carnaval* cross-dressing, the *travestis* (transvestites) of Brazil view transvestism as an identity and a designation that pervades every aspect of their lives. Although the clinical literature emphasizes that transvestites do not live continuously in the cross-gender role, and that their cross-dressing is periodic and fetishistic (Docter 1988:39; Docter and Prince 1997), for the *travestis* of Brazil, transvestism appears to be enduring—typically lifelong.

Travestis in Brazil, as in other cultures, are marked by an exaggerated femininity in both dress and makeup (Kulick 1998). They come almost exclusively from the poorest segments of Brazilian society, but there is little toleration for them in either the *favelas* (shantytowns) or the traditional, low-income suburban areas. Thus, as they begin to cross the lines of gender, most leave behind family and friends, emigrating to Rio de Janeiro, São Paulo, and other large cities into districts where

> a mixture of socially marginal and often illegal activities creates not only a kind of moral region but a moral anonymity in which the traditional values of Brazilian society cease to function. Within this world (which is also the world of female prostitution, drug trafficking, homosexuality, and the more sporadic prostitution of the *miches* [male prostitutes]), given pervasive prejudice and discrimination, almost no options other than prostitution are open to the *travesti* for earning a living; as a result, almost all *travestis* quickly become involved in prostitution as their primary activity (Daniel and Parker 1993:91).

Most transvestites live in close proximity to each other, in the rundown sections of the *asfalto* where rents are extremely low. During the course of the fieldwork for this study, for example, the authors visited some of the residences of the transvestites. For several, their apartments were eight-foot by ten-foot rooms, each the size of a prison cell, in a building that had been converted from nineteenth-century slave quarters.

Transvestites always dress as women, and when referring to one another, they use such pronouns as "her" and "she." Many use drugs, and because of their involvement in street prostitution, they are regularly exposed to both violence and a full range of sexually transmitted diseases, including HIV and AIDS. For example, among 57 drug-using transvestites engaging in prostitution in Rome (the great majority of whom had emigrated from Brazil), the overall prevalence of HIV was 74 percent (Gattari et al. 1992). Studies conducted in various parts of Brazil over the past ten years also reflect high rates of HIV seropositivity among transvestite sex workers. Among 37 transvestites tested in São Paulo during 1988, 62 percent were found to be HIV positive (Suleiman et al. 1989), and among 112 transvestites contacted four years later, 60.7 percent tested positive (Grandi et al. 1993).

In Rio de Janeiro, it is estimated that there are at least 2,000 transvestites, 80 percent of whom support themselves through prostitution. Within this context, the balance of this chapter examines aspects of the subculture of male transvestite sex workers in Rio de Janeiro, with a particular focus on their drug-using and sexual risk behaviors.

The Culture of *Travestismo* in Rio De Janeiro

The qualitative and quantitative data reported here on *travestismo* (transvestism) and *travestis* (transvestites) in Rio de Janeiro were collected as part of the larger HIV/AIDS prevention initiative described earlier in Chapters 3 and 4. A total of 1,644 individuals had been recruited into the project, of whom 100 were male transvestite sex workers. Data collection on the *travestis* occurred in three phases (1) street recruitment as part of the overall project outreach and intervention effort, (2) numerous focus groups, and (3) participant observation.

Street Recruitment

Two cohorts of male transvestite prostitutes were sampled from the *asfalto*. The first (N=52) were recruited from the "Lapa" and "Copacabana" neighborhoods of Rio de Janeiro. Lapa is a downtown section of the city described in guide books as an inner residential area, with some sections having numerous strip clubs and cheap hotels, many of which are considered "hot pillow establishments" (Box 1994:371; Box 1997:400). It is an old Bohemian area, famous in the past for its night life. However, as drug users, prostitutes, and transvestites began moving into Lapa and establishing themselves, the area began to deteriorate. Late at night, along such thoroughfares as Mem de Sá and Riachuelo, transvestite prostitutes can be observed soliciting their clientele. In fact, the particular street or boulevard they are soliciting generally dictates how much and what kind of clothing they will be wearing. Along some of the more heavily traveled thoroughfares, for example, most of the transvestites observed are scantily covered, dressed in tight skirts and halter tops. Several blocks further into Lapa, most are topless, clearly displaying their hormone or silicone enhanced breasts. By the parks in Lapa, some transvestites are modestly dressed in loose skirts, which they raise to display their penises as potential clients walk or drive by.

Copacabana, famous since the 1920s as a flamboyant ocean resort, is a narrow, curving expanse covering just over four square kilometers. It is the most populous community in Rio de Janeiro, and its 250,000 residents make it one of the most densely inhabited areas of the world. High-rise apartments and hotels line the elite and expensive beach-front Avenida Atlântica, but behind it are 109 narrow streets and alleyways that mark a neighborhood in which as many as ten people are often crammed into small, two-bedroom apartments. Although prostitutes are active on many streets in Copacabana, including "Posto 6" and Rua Rainha Eliza-beth, late at night transvestites can be found concentrated on an easterly segment of Avenida Atlântica, not too distant from the world-renowned, five-star Hotel Meridien. Most stand in the streets waving at motorists, while others patrol the sidewalk cafes.

The second cohort (N=48) of transvestites was sampled from a distant suburb of Rio de Janeiro known as *Baixada fluminense*, an area containing more than 2.6 million persons, the majority of whom were living in abject poverty. The *baixada* is considered one of the poorest areas of Brazil, with infant mortality rates and the incidence of infectious diseases five times higher than in Rio de Janeiro. Lacking a sewerage disposal system and potable drinking water, and awash in garbage, *Baixada fluminense* is con-sidered a public health disaster where tetanus, typhoid, meningitis, and a variety of intestinal infections are commonplace, especially among chil-dren (Taylor 1994). Yet surprisingly, rates of HIV infection are found to be lower in the *baixada* than in the downtown sections of Rio de Janeiro (Telles et al. 1996).

Initially, the recruitment of male transvestite sex workers was con-ducted by outreach workers, on a one-night-a-week basis. Because trans-vestites are highly reviled in Rio de Janeiro and are frequently the targets of violence, outreach workers typically operated in pairs for the sake of their own personal safety.[1] Contacts were made on the street, and in the bars, strip clubs, hotels, and rooming houses frequented by transvestites. Success at recruitment was limited, however, for a variety of reasons. First, the great majority of the transvestites contacted began "working" quite late in the night, and slept most of the day, and as such were un-willing to participate in the study during the project's operating hours. Second, the travel stipend paid to project clients was R$10 in Brazilian currency (about U.S.$10), for each visit and was considered too low to en-tice many transvestite sex workers to make the trip. For those coming from *Baixada fluminense*, the commute was nearly two hours by bus. Third, many were either afraid of being tested for HIV, or already knew their HIV status. Finally, because of widespread discrimination against transvestites, many were suspicious of any university-based project, including this one.

As an alternative to traditional outreach techniques, two additional procedures were implemented. Since the latex condoms available in Rio de Janeiro are expensive and sometimes of low quality, transvestite recruits were promised 40 U.S.-made condoms in addition to the regular travel stipend when they appeared at the project office. Moreover, transvestite key informants from local organizations were retained as part-time outreach workers. These strategies resulted in the recruitment of 52 transvestite sex workers from Lapa and Copacabana, and 48 from *Baixada fluminense*.

Once contacted in the field, all project clients were either transported to, or given directions to, the project assessment center, located in the São Cristóvão section of Rio de Janeiro. All interviewing, drawing of blood for HIV testing, pretest and posttest counseling, and AIDS prevention training were conducted at this center.

Focus Groups

Because the standardized Risk Behavior Assessment (RBA) instrument designed for the 23 Cooperative Agreement sites was primarily for injection drug users, few questions related to sexual risks of a historical nature, and none of the questions targeted the special risks associated with male transvestite sex work. Furthermore, the RBA had not been designed to elicit information about cultural and lifestyle issues. As a result, the authors conducted numerous focus groups, each containing five to seven transvestites. Topics included their views of prostitution and transvestism, employment patterns, sexual activities, condom use, drug use, and mechanisms of feminization.

Participant Observation

In an effort to better understand the patterns of behavior of male transvestite sex workers in Rio de Janeiro, the authors made a number of trips to the field areas where transvestites typically solicit their clients. These visits were conducted during the hours that the transvestites worked. Observations focused primarily on how transvestites congregated in the streets and how they solicited clients. In addition, the authors toured transvestite working and living areas with the director of ASTRAL (Asso-

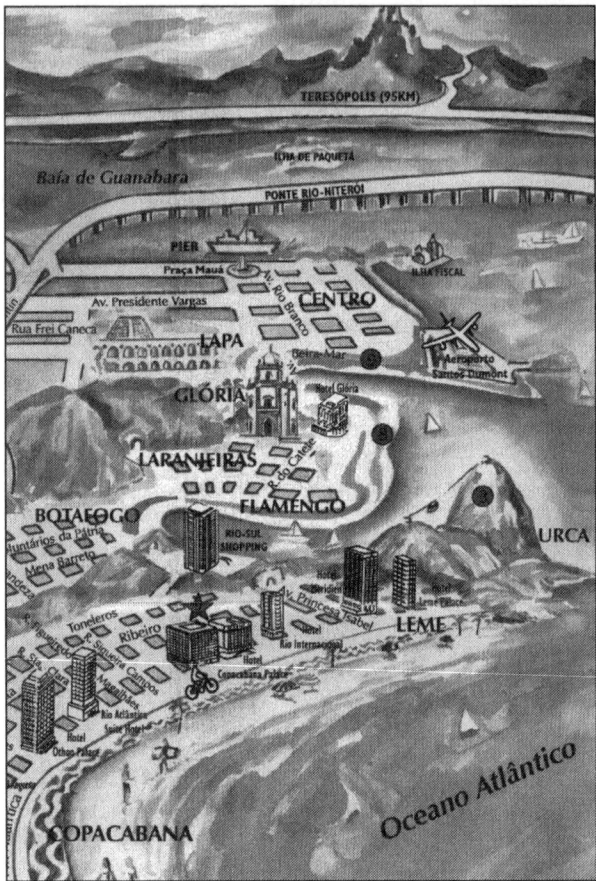

MAP 6.2   Rio de Janeiro Field Areas

ciation for Transvestites and the Liberated), a local organization established to promote safe sex among male transvestite sex workers and their
clients.

Drug Use, Sexual Behavior, and HIV/AIDS

Because the lifestyles and patterns of sexual behavior appear to be similar among both samples of the male transvestite sex workers recruited
into this study, the data for each of the two cohorts are presented aggre-
gately. As illustrated in Table 6.1, the transvestites sampled were young,
with a median age of 26 years. The overwhelming majority had minimal
education, with only 22 percent completing more than eight years of

TABLE 6.1   Demographic Characteristics of 100 Male Transvestite Sex Workers, Rio de Janeiro, Brazil

Age at Interview	
18–24	34.0%
25–34	51.0%
35+	15.0%
Median	26.0
Race/Ethnicity	
Black	32.0%
White	38.0%
Multiracial	30.0%
Education	
Less than 8 years	78.0%
More than 8 years	22.0%
*Monthly Income**	
Less than $100	16.0%
$101–$300	32.0%
$301–$600	29.0%
$601–$1,000	14.0%
$1001+	7.0%
Don't Know	2.0%

*Income data were collected as number of minimum wages, then converted into U.S. dollars using an average minimum salary of R$100 per month at an exchange or 1:1.

school. Further, white, black (Afro-Brazilian), and multiracial (*mulato, pardo,* and *moreno*) individuals were evenly represented in the sample. The data in Table 6.1 also suggest that the earnings of these transvestites were not high. The median monthly income of the sample was U.S. $450.00, which is equivalent to the salary of a part-time secretary or interviewer in Brazil. And although the data are not delineated in Table 6.1, four-fifths of the sample reported earnings through prostitution during the 30-day period prior to interview, with the remaining 20 percent having income from other illegal activities, selling/trading goods, odd jobs, and/or friends and relatives.

Table 6.2 indicates that almost all of the transvestites had histories of alcohol use (91%), and that the majority had some experience with both marijuana (61%) and cocaine (76%). Other drugs, such as heroin, amphetamines, and hallucinogens were not reported because they are generally unavailable in Rio de Janeiro. In terms of sequential patterns of drug use

TABLE 6.3   Sexual Behavior of 100 Male Transvestite Sex Workers, Rio de Janeiro, Brazil

Number of Sexual Partners*	
Fewer than 10	34.0%
10–30	16.0%
31+	50.0%
Unprotected Insertive Anal Sex*	13.0%
Unprotected Receptive Anal Sex*	32.0%
Cocaine Use during Sex*	31.0%
Ever Traded Sex for Drugs	29.0%
STD History	39.0%

*Reference period is last 30 days prior to interview.

TABLE 6.4   Significant Predictors of HIV Infection for 100 Male Transvestite Sex Workers, Rio de Janeiro, Brazil

	Regression Coefficient	*Odds Ratio*	*95% C.I.*
Sample*	-2.128	.119	(.03, .43)
Age*	1.661	5.267	(1.51, 18.3)
Education*	-1.750	.174	(.04, .81)
Drug Injection History*	2.458	11.682	(1.07, 128.12)
Unprotected Insertive Anal Sex*	2.160	8.670	(1.21, 62.2)

*Reference category for sample is sample 1; reference category for education is less than 8 years of school; reference category for injection history is no; reference category for unprotected insertive anal sex is no.

icantly related to HIV seropositivity included older age, lower education, having ever injected drugs, and having had unprotected insertive anal sex. Surprisingly, none of the other variables in the model, including unprotected receptive anal sex, appeared to relate to serostatus.

Because this project counted among its aims the reassessment of HIV risk behaviors levels among clients who participated in the intervention, an attempt was made to recontact the 100 participants at three months after the baseline interview. And because many of the recruitment difficulties noted earlier in this book persisted into the follow-up phase of the project, only 39 of the participants who were relocated agreed to be reinterviewed. When examining risk behaviors at follow-up, no changes were apparent on any of the sexual behavior dimensions. In other words, participants neither decreased the number of sexual partners, modified the types of sexual activities engaged in, nor increased condom use in response to the intervention.

Feminization

Given that the male transvestites contacted as part of the project were active sex workers, exchanged sex for drugs and/or money, had numerous sex partners (a median of 30 in the past 30 days), histories of sexually transmitted diseases, and participated in both receptive and insertive anal sex, it is not surprising that almost half tested positive for antibodies to HIV. Focus group data offered further insights into why these rates were so high. During these sessions participants described the feminization process using repeated silicone injections, a virtually unstudied potential risk factor for HIV transmission among male transvestites (see Goihman et al. 1994). The focus group data suggested that the use of silicone was widespread among the 100 clients recruited into the project. It was reported that the great majority of the transvestites in Rio de Janeiro undergo silicone injections to shape their bodies. These "beauty treatments," as the clients referred to them, are done by other "experienced" transvestites who are too old to support themselves as street prostitutes. The injection equipment was typically shared by several transvestites, with less than adequate cleaning between each use. Industrial quality silicone was most commonly used because it could be purchased by the gallon at a relatively cheap price. Numerous injections, sometimes more than 70 punctures, were required to accomplish each individual body shape. Since this was a painful process, it was common for transvestites to be under the influence of alcohol and/or drugs during the process. The injected liquid silicone had a tendency to dislodge after a few months, and thus, new injections were required periodically to reshape certain parts of the body. Moreover, infections were common after such procedures and often plastic surgery was the only recourse to remove the dislodged silicone.

The high rate of HIV infection observed among male transvestite sex workers demonstrates the need to include this population in both outreach and intervention efforts. Prevention/intervention initiatives need to be designed to address specific risk factors of this vulnerable population. Despite these obvious facts, many transvestites' lifestyle issues continue to be neglected by traditional and current AIDS prevention campaigns possibly due to the low status accorded them by Brazilian society.

The general lack of insight into the role of the *travestis* as they define it further attests to the marginalization of the population. For example, focus group data indicate that the *travestis* of Rio de Janeiro, contrary to much of the literature on transvestism, do not consider themselves to be heterosexual. Although they report feeling sexually attracted to men, they do not identify themselves as either *women* or *male homosexuals.* Rather, they view themselves as having a separate gender identity, which they designate as "transvestite." Furthermore, unlike gay men, transvestites do not have a sexual interest in male homosexuals, but to men "who are normally attracted to women."

Ideally, transvestites wish their sex partners to look at them as women, to take the active role in anal intercourse, and to ignore the transvestite's masculine genitalia during sex. Although transvestites are attempting to appear as women, it is not their intent to "pass" as women. At the same time, a transvestite typically keeps "her" penis hidden from her insertive partners during sexual intercourse through special clothes or posture. However, this act of "hiding" is more apt to take place when a transvestite sex worker is engaging in sexual activity with clients as opposed to their steady partners. Playing the active role in a sexual encounter is considered by many participants to be a violation of their "ideal sexuality," although many engaged in this behavior in order to satisfy their clientele. However, although transvestites dress as, and wish to be viewed as women by their partners, many express a special repugnance for the vagina and believe transsexual surgery to be nonsensical.

Postscript

An effective AIDS prevention initiative targeting this population must take these notions of gender identity and sexuality into account, and include the following strategies. First, although transvestite sex workers are aware of the importance of condoms during anal sex, few actually use them. Not only are condoms generally unavailable, but their clients are often unwilling to use them. As such, not only must there be greater availability of condoms, but mechanisms to teach transvestites how to negotiate condom use with clients. Condom negotiation and empowerment techniques have long since been a part of risk reduction initiatives for women, but because transvestites are typically looked upon as "men," this aspect of prevention programming is typically forgotten.

Second, the authors were the first people to introduce the female condom to Brazilian transvestites (Inciardi and Surratt 1995, 1996). Pilot work determined that not only did transvestite sex workers consider the female condom to be an acceptable method of HIV risk reduction during anal sex, but also that they liked it and were willing and eager to use it.

As such, female condom distribution and instruction in its use would appear to be a crucial part of AIDS prevention for this population.

Third, there is the problem of the repeated use of contaminated needles and syringes during silicone injections. This is not a topic that is addressed in contemporary AIDS prevention programs. Although the cleaning of injection paraphernalia is discussed with drug users, more general HIV prevention discussions bypass the topic. In this regard, information about the hazards associated with using potentially infected needles must be provided not only to transvestite sex workers, but also to the other members of their subculture who actually administer the injections.

Note

1. During September and October of 1994, just after the recruitment of transvestites was initiated, 20 were found murdered, presumably at the hands of police death squads.

7

Street Children and
the Drugs/AIDS Connection

During the mid-1990s, the United Nations Center for Human Rights estimated that by the beginning of the twenty-first century half of the world's population will be under 25 years of age and located in cities, and that significant numbers will be living in poverty (UNICEF 1996a). The United Nations also estimated that by the year 2000 there would be almost 250 million more urban children in the 5- to 19-year-old age cohort than there were in the mid-1980s; that more than 90 percent of these youths would be living in developing nations; and that by the year 2020 there would be some 100 million indigent urban minors in Latin America alone. It is likely, furthermore, that many of these children will be living in the streets (UNICEF 1996b).

The use of the street as a place to live and/or work is not unknown to most industrial economies, but the presence of vast numbers of unsupervised and unprotected children is a phenomenon that is visible only in developing nations, and particularly in Latin America (Rizzini and Lusk 1995; Lusk 1989). Estimates of the number of street children throughout Central and South America vary widely, but the United Nations Children's Fund figure of 40 million is the most generally accepted (UNICEF 1996b). Many of these youths are exploited and abused, and because of their pariah status in the eyes of the public they are referred to with a variety of disapproving appellations—*gamines* (urchins) and *chinches* in Colombia, *pajaros fruteros* in Peru, and *marginais* (nonessentials or criminals), *pivetes* (little farts), and *abandonados* (children who have nowhere else to go) in Brazil. And in few places are the street children more visible, and reviled, than in Brazil.

The Southeastern region of Brazil, where São Paulo and Rio de Janeiro are situated, is the most heavily populated section of the country. It is estimated that in metropolitan Rio de Janeiro and São Paulo alone there are several million children living in extreme poverty. And it is this destitution that drives children to the streets in an attempt to survive.

Meninos de Rua

Throughout Latin America, *meninos de rua* (in Brazilian Portuguese) or *niños de la calle* (in Spanish) represent the new face of child labor—youths working in the urban informal sector. Their occupations range from shining shoes and selling cigarettes, flowers, newspapers or chewing gum to hauling garbage, drug trafficking, petty theft, street robberies, and prostitution.

The existence of street children in the large metropolitan areas of Brazil is not particularly new. The international media began to document the condition of large numbers of Brazilian street children as early as the 1970s. Despite the significant media attention over the past 15 to 20 years, however, much remains unknown about their daily lives and activities. In fact, even approximating the actual size of the population of street children has proven difficult. Estimates of their numbers in Brazil have ranged from 7 to 17 million, but more informed assessments suggest that between 7 and 8 million children, ages 5 to 18, live and/or work on the streets of urban Brazil. While the vast majority of street children are boys, Brazilian government estimates put the number of street girls at approximately 800,000, with almost two-thirds of them working as prostitutes in various parts of the country (Barker 1992).

Part of the problem in estimating the number of street children lies in the distinction between what are known as "children *on* the street" and "children *of* the street" (Campos, et al. 1994; Lusk 1989). Children *on* the street work in informal sector occupations in order to supplement the family income, but return home at night to sleep. These children typically reside in households headed by impoverished, single women and spend most of the day and night in the street selling candy or gum, guarding cars, shining shoes, or carrying groceries.

By contrast, children *of* the street have oftentimes completely severed ties with their families. They seemingly choose to leave homes where hunger, neglect, and exploitation are commonplace, making life on the street preferable. A very small number of children actually live full time in the streets, often engaging in illegal activities in order to survive. In fact, children *of* the street are more typically associated with drug sales, petty theft, prostitution, and gang activity. Younger children often begin their careers on the street by begging, but rely increasingly on crime to support themselves as they age and become less successful at panhandling. Young street girls commonly use prostitution as a way of supporting themselves.

As indicated in Table 7.1, the United Nations Children's Fund estimates that the number of "working children" (children *on* the street) and

TABLE 7.1 "Working Children" and "Street Children" in
Selected Latin American and Caribbean Nations

Country	Working Children	Street Children
Argentina	2.35 million	20,000*
Bolivia	72,000	200
Brazil	7.4 million	8 million[†]
Costa Rica	53,000	5,300
Ecuador	1 million	4,000
El Salvador	231,000	10,000
Guatemala	1.62 million	1,000[††]
Haiti	120,000	10,000
Honduras	275,000	800
Mexico	10 million	250,000

*Includes Buenos Aires only.
[†]May include children working, but not living, on the street.
[††]Include Guatemala City only.
SOURCE: UNICEF, Regional Office for Latin America, Bogota.

"street children" (children *of* the street) throughout Latin America total as many as 40 million.

As the number of street children and their related criminal activity continue to grow, so does public opposition to their presence. Over the past twenty or so years, public opinion has shifted dramatically. Youngsters who were once looked upon as deserving of compassion and sympathy are now viewed at best as a nuisance, and at worst as a danger to public safety—future criminals who ought to be locked up. Although popular views characterize these children as delinquents and thieves, perhaps Nancy Scheper-Hughes most accurately described street youths in modern Brazil as simply "poor children in the wrong place" (Scheper-Hughes and Hoffman 1994). Perhaps it was this sentiment that enabled the Brazilian National Congress to pass the Child and Adolescent Act in 1990. This statute was designed to reform the legal status of children in Brazil and to create councils that would act as children's rights advocates, with an eye toward integrating impoverished children into the larger society. However, negative attitudes toward street children by the Brazilian people prevail and public resistance to such reforms continues to frustrate attempts to implement the statute.

The Children of the *Favelas*

Important to understanding the presence of large numbers of street children in Latin America in general, and in Brazil in particular, is a comprehension of the nature of primate cities and what life is like in the thousands of primate city shantytowns.

Most developing countries contain one or more "primate cities," urban areas that grow in population and influence far beyond the other cities in the region or nation. In many Latin American countries, and in other developing nations as well, the largest cities may have several times the combined populations of the next two or three urban areas and may also have a significant share of the national population. Mexico City's population of 16 million, for example, accounts for 20 percent of the nation's population, while other cities are considerably smaller: Guadalajara (1.6 million), Monterrey (1.1 million), and Puebla de Zaragoza (1.1 million). Similarly, the populations of Brazil's two largest cities—São Paulo and Rio de Janeiro—combine to account for some 16 percent of the national population.

Primate cities typically are located on the coast or in other areas close to transportation routes, since many were political and economic centers when under colonial rule. The orientation of such cities had been toward supplying the developed nations with raw materials and other goods, rather than toward the urban areas and hinterlands of their own country.

Among the greatest difficulties experienced by these cities in Latin America are those of stimulating industrialization and providing employment. People who move into these urban locales do so, not because of the employment opportunities the cities provide, but because the living conditions in rural areas seem so much worse. Previous research has suggested that rural populations have been "forced" to relocate because of increasing agricultural density and the inability of the land to support its people (Firebaugh 1979). Rural to urban migrants believe that the cities offer a better life and at least the hope for employment. Some do find work in small enterprises, but the lack of sophisticated technology and industrial production methods does not provide for the large pool of unskilled labor that characterized the Western industrial revolution. As a result, the unemployment rates in the cities of many developing nations often exceed 25 percent of the labor force.

Common features of the primate city landscape are the sections comprised of shanties, shacks, and makeshift huts inhabited by those who have no other shelter. Known as *barriadas* in Peru, *ranchos* in Venezuela, *villas miserias* in Argentina, or as described earlier in Chapter 4, *favelas* in Brazil, these squatter settlements have been estimated to house as much as one-third of the urban population (Butterworth and Chance 1981:151–157). Mexico City has some 4 million squatters, Calcutta has 2 million, and Rio de Janeiro has more than 1 million.

Favelas have been a feature of urban Brazil for generations (Freyre 1986). *Favela* in Brazilian Portuguese means "slum." Yet it is a particular type of slum that takes its name from *Morro da Favela*, a hill near Rio de Janeiro where the first one appeared in the late 1880s. In 1963, the noted journalist and biographer John Dos Passos commented:

> In Rio—this was in 1948—there were said to be three hundred thousand people living in *favelas*. Today there are nearer a million. You come on *favelas* in the most unexpected places. In Copacabana a few minutes walk from the hotels and the splendid white apartment houses and the well kept magnificent beaches you find a whole hillside of *favelas* overlooking the lake and the Jockey Club. In the center of Rio a few steps from the Avenida Rio Branco on the hill behind one of the most fashionable churches you come suddenly into a tropical jungle town (Dos Passos 1963:31).

Similarly, in 1966 noted travel writer John Gunther described Rio's *favelas* as "vertical" in character—since they were situated on hillsides:

> This came about partly because much of the land in Rio is too steep for normal building purposes and, when urbanization began on a serious scale, speculators let the hills alone. So the squatters swarmed to the cliffs, scraped off plots from jungle shrubbery, and built their miserable huts out of tin cans, hunks of stone, and cardboard, on the sharpest slopes. The irony is that they now have the best views in the city. But there are no amenities whatever, not even water or a postal service. Filth and flies are everywhere. Dogs howl, and children drip with slime (Gunther 1966:72).

The *favelas* situated on the hillsides of Rio de Janeiro are the best known and most notorious. They began to appear at the end of the nineteenth century, and spread rapidly after 1930 as shelters for newly arriving migrants (Burns 1980:569). Fleeing regions hard-hit by drought and unemployment, rural Brazilians thronged to the *cidade maravilhosa*, the "marvelous city" of Rio de Janeiro, lured by its illusionary riches. And there has been a steady stream even since. At the close of the 1980s, it was estimated that some 1,500 *favelados* were arriving each day (Archambault 1989). Although the number of new arrivals had declined significantly by the close of the 1990s, the *favelas* nevertheless continue to expand.

Little has changed since Dos Passos and Gunther made their observations decades ago, although "children dripping with slime" was clearly a journalist's overstatement. In the great majority of the *favelas*, migrants from all over Brazil have recreated a semirural way of life, in neighborhoods with names that often reflect a bittersweet Brazilian humor—*Morro da Esperança* (Hill of Hope), *Chácara do Céu* (Sky Gardens), and *Nova Brasília* (New Brasília). In Rio de Janeiro, the *favelas* have been estimated by Brazil's Municipal Planning Institute to number 545 and house more than 1 million persons—some 14 percent of the city's population (Loveman 1991). As noted earlier in Chapter 4, there is disease, drug use, and prostitution, and virtually no medical or social services in these communities (Guillermoprieto 1990; Rambali 1993). Within such a setting, it is no wonder that so many children retreat from the *favelas* to the streets—in Rio de Janeiro, São Paulo, Belo Horizonte, Porto Alegre, Santos, Fortaleza, Recife, and other Brazilian cities. And in Rio, a city where street children have received considerable media attention, they withdraw from the *favelas* to Copacabana, Ipanema, Leblon, Lapa, Botafogo, Tijuca, and other sections of the "asphalt city." The total number of street youths in Rio de Janeiro has been the topic of considerable media conjecture and exaggeration, with some estimates as high 1 million. Local public health officials put the number of "children *of* the street" at 2,000 to 3,000 (*Facts on File* 1996), which still is a major social problem.

Drug Use among Street Youths

Anecdotal accounts of drug abuse among street youths in Brazil are commonplace. Numerous media stories have reported the widespread use of inhalants (such as glue; gasoline; lighter fluid; *bim* B, a mixture of ethyl alcohol, sugar and benzene), marijuana and cocaine, and Valium among street children in Rio de Janeiro (Brookes 1991; Larmer 1992). Also common is the use of coca paste and Rohypnol.

Common not only in the drug-using communities of Brazil, but also in those of Colombia, Bolivia, Venezuela, Ecuador, and Peru, is the use of coca paste, known to most South Americans as *basuco, susuko, pasta básica de cocaína, pasta de coca,* or just simply *pasta* (Jeri 1984). Perhaps best known as *basuco,* coca paste is one of the intermediate products in the processing of the coca leaf into cocaine. It is typically smoked straight, or in cigarettes mixed with either tobacco or marijuana.

The smoking of coca paste became popular in South America beginning in the early 1970s. It was readily available, inexpensive, had a high cocaine content, and was absorbed quickly. As the phenomenon was studied, however, it was quickly realized that paste smoking was far more serious than any other form of cocaine use. In addition to cocaine, paste contains traces of all the chemicals used to initially process the coca leaves—kerosene, sulfuric acid, methanol, benzoic acid, and the oxidized products of these solvents, plus any number of other alkaloids that are present in the coca leaf (Almeida 1978).

When the smoking of paste was first noted in South America it seemed to be restricted to the coca processing regions of Bolivia, Colombia, Ecuador, and Peru, appealing primarily to street children and low-income groups due to its cheap price when compared with that of refined cocaine (Jeri et al. 1976). By the early 1980s, however, it had spread to other South American nations, including Brazil, to numerous segments of the social strata, and throughout the decade paste smoking further expanded to become a major drug problem for much of South America.[1] Among the Rio street youth of the 1990s, the smoking of coca pasta remained an enduring problem.

By contrast, Rohypnol is a legal drug in Brazil, readily available in pharmacies in many parts of the world. Also known by its generic name, flunitrazepam, Rohypnol is a benzodiazepine drug having anticonvulsant and sedative effects, slowing psychomotor performance, and inducing muscle relaxation and sleep. It is used for the short-term treatment of insomnia. However, its use can lead to the development of physical and psychic dependence, with the risk of addiction increasing with dose and duration of use (Saum and Inciardi 1997).

Rohypnol is similar to Valium, but ten times as potent. It was first introduced in the 1970s, and is legally available throughout Europe and Latin America. Since the 1980s it has been used to counter some of the negative side effects of cocaine abuse. In addition, combining Rohypnol with alcohol, cocaine, or marijuana reportedly produces a fast "hit" followed by a mellow state that lasts for several hours.

Many street youths in Rio de Janeiro see their use of inhalants, coca paste, marijuana, Rohypnol, and other drugs as an escape—a way to dull their hunger and facilitate acts of prostitution and other crimes (Barker 1992; Vasconcelos 1990). And as one young female prostitute observed:

> When I was prostituting at the boarding house, my father would go there and want to pay me to have sex with him. I would never do it and every time he would leave, I would smoke a lot of marijuana to try and forget the things that he would say (Vasconcelos 1990).

Indeed, it has been observed that drug use by street children is a nearly universal phenomenon because these youths are confronted with the harsh realities of street life on a daily basis (Lusk 1989). Given that drug abuse among youths has emerged as a concomitant of life on the streets, the paucity of scientific studies that have examined this and other related topics among street children in Brazil is troubling.

Although previous research on drug use among street children is limited, existing studies have found rates of use to be high. A survey among 119 street children in São Paulo, for example, classified 45 percent as heavy drug users, indicating the use of up to three drugs a day (Dimenstein 1991). In a study of street youths in Belo Horizonte, a city of 2 million people some 452 kilometers northeast of Rio de Janeiro, 84 percent of the children living full time in the street had histories of illegal drug use, 10.6 percent reported injection drug use, and 83.5 percent were sexually active (Campos, et al. 1994). Additionally, in an earlier study involving this same sample, 82.6 percent reported having had sex while under the influence of drugs and/or alcohol. In comparison, of the working but "home-based" children interviewed, only 25 percent had histories of illegal drug use and *none* reported the use of injection drugs (Campos et al. 1992). A similar study supported these findings by reporting higher rates of drug use among "street-based" youth than "home-based" youth, 76.9 percent versus 29.1 percent, and earlier onset of drug use—9.8 years versus 11.2 years (Pinto et al. 1992). Moreover, a 1992 study of 98 street children in Rio de Janeiro found that 90.8 percent believed drug abuse to be a problem in the community and 38.8 percent stated that drug use was a personal problem for them (Eisenstein and De Aquino 1992). The most commonly used drugs among these children were glue (13.3%), marijuana (13.3%), alcohol/tobacco (12.2%), and cocaine (11.2%). Nearly 70 percent of this sample refused to respond to questions about injection drug use.

The most in-depth study of drug use among street youths was conducted in 1992 by the Guidance Center on Drugs and the Treatment of Drug Addicts of the University of Brasília (De Paula 1992). The research sampled 150 males ages 10 to 17 in Ceilândia, one of Brasília's satellite cities, and examined three groups of street children—youths with no school or family ties, youths receiving assistance from social welfare institutions (typically delinquents), and youths enrolled in local schools. The data indicated that a full 100 percent of the street youths interviewed used drugs. Solvents and inhalants, typically cobbler's glue, were the most commonly used. "Frequent use," defined as daily or several times a week, was found among 88 percent of the entire sample, and among 72 percent of those in social welfare institutions. In addition, 32 percent of the youths reported the use of marijuana and/or cocaine. The latter drugs are purchased from local dealers, while the inhalants can be obtained legally in a variety of places.

The fact that solvents and inhalants are the drugs most frequently used by street youths was not an unanticipated finding of the Brasília study, because prior studies have found these drugs to be common among other youth populations as well. In a study of 1,836 São Paulo students (ages 9 to 18 years) from low socioeconomic backgrounds, 24 percent reported lifetime use of inhalants and 4.9 percent reported use in the last 30 days (Carlini-Cotrim and Carlini 1988). Moreover, in a ten-city survey of 16,300 Brazilian public school students 26.2 percent reported lifetime use of psychotropic drugs—typically solvents and inhalants (Carlini and Carlini-Cotrim 1993).

Sex and HIV Risks

Regardless of whether they reported any use of illegal drugs, street children have frequently reported engaging in risky sexual behaviors. Street studies in Rio de Janeiro have concluded that a "second shift" of children are visible on the streets at night. Unlike their daytime counterparts, these "second shift" children tend to be older and are more likely to be female. Among them, prostitution is frequent by both boys and girls (Lusk 1989). A 1992 study of 62 children found that 48.4 percent had engaged in sex, 60 percent with adult men, 16.6 percent reported sex for money, but only 33.3 percent reported any use of condoms (Campos, et al. 1994).

In addition to solicitation for prostitution, many street children have reported incidents of rape. Scheper-Hughes and Hoffman (1994) observed that street girls and boys are frequently raped by police and others. Surprisingly, however, the perpetrators are not always male. Vasconcelos (1990) noted that older street girls will sometimes force younger girls to have sex with them, thereby continuing the cycle of violence of which they too have been victims. Of the 98 street children interviewed by Eisenstein and De Aquino (1992), 53.1 percent were sexually active and 44.9 percent reported being forced to have sex. Similarly, a survey of 52 HIV seropositive street youths under age 16 in Rio de Janeiro found that 28 percent had had anal intercourse, presumably forced. Of those ages 7 to 12, 63 percent had had anal intercourse and 57 percent had been forced to have anal intercourse by older street children (Van Buuren and Bezerra 1992).

Although this type of sexual violence appears to be common, it is not always necessary. Many street children use sex as a way to gain affection and attention (Scheper-Hughes and Hoffman 1994). For this reason, younger girls at times voluntarily seek sexual contact with older girls (Vasconcelos 1990). Sexual activity among boys is also relatively common. Some 21 percent of street boys interviewed in a 1991 study reported same-sex anal intercourse (Ude et al. 1991). Heterosexual anal intercourse was reported by 43 percent of these same respondents.

Despite high rates of sexual activity among street children, attitudes regarding condom use are for the most part negative and usage rates are low. Various studies have reported the proportion of sexually active street children having ever used condoms to be in the range of 8.2 percent to 33.3 percent (Campos, et al. 1994; Eisenstein and de Aquino 1992; Raffaelli et al. 1992; Ude et al. 1991).

Risk of exposure to HIV is rapidly becoming an area of concern because of the large number of street youths engaging in unprotected sexual acts, both remunerated and nonremunerated. On the whole, the

World Health Organization reckons that there are between 50,000 and 100,000 HIV positive children and adolescents in Brazil. Going further, it has also been estimated that between 1 percent and 2 percent of Brazil's population of 7 to 8 million street children, or between 70,000 and 110,000 individuals, are HIV positive. A study in 1987–1988 at the FUNBEM Hospital in Rio de Janeiro found that among 3,389 street children, 50 (1.5%) were HIV positive (Eisenstein 1993). However, a more recent study conducted between May 1991 and January 1994 found that of 126 street children interviewed and tested, 94 percent reported HIV risk behaviors, and 6 percent were HIV seropositive (Adams et al. 1994).

Violence Against Street Children

Street children throughout Latin America are viewed by many police groups, merchants, and other citizens as undesirable, pariah populations (Thomas 1995:88–89). In Brazil, they are targets of fear, and are seen by the upper classes and the political right wing as being:

> . . . a blemish on the urban landscape and a reminder that all is not well in the country. Unwanted and considered human waste, these ubiquitous tattered, mainly black children and adolescents evoke strong and contradictory emotions of fear, aversion, pity and anger in those who view their neighborhood streets, boulevards and squares as "private places" under siege (Scheper-Hughes and Hoffman 1994:23).

Because of their drug use, predatory crimes, and general unacceptability on urban thoroughfares, street children have frequently been the targets of local vigilante groups, drug gangs, and police "death squads."

Perhaps most notorious have been the death squads, which initially appeared in Brazil in 1968, and primarily in Rio de Janeiro, at first to avenge the terrorist murder of a well-known police officer. The death squads proliferated during the years of Brazil's military rule, which ended in 1985. As the killings spread, political and community leaders were often targeted, and the victims were easily recognized. Their hands were always tied behind their backs, their tongues cut out, and a crudely drawn skull and crossbones were left on the corpse with the initials "E.M."—"Esquadrão de Morte"—appended.

News reports have suggested that there are many such police assassination squads in Latin America (Barker 1992). Guatemala had its *La Mano Blanco* (The White Hand); Argentina its Anti-Communist Alliance; the Dominican Republic its *La Banda* gang; and in Brazil, Paraguay, Honduras, and El Salvador simply *Esquadrão de Morte* or *Esquadron de Muerte*

"Death Squad." All were organized, but unofficial, police vigilante organizations established with the aim not only of preserving their respective political regimes through selective political murders, but also of eliminating those viewed by the police as "undesirables"—trade unionists, drug dealers, thieves, and other criminals, and not surprisingly, street children.

Many of the death squads still exist, particularly in Brazil, and street children are common victims. Because they survive, in part, through prostitution and crime, they have become the targets of retributive violence by police death squads and merchants' vigilante groups (Martins 1992). Considered to be bad for business, store owners hire off-duty police officers or professional killers to eliminate the "disposable children." Their elimination is also seen as a mechanism of "social cleansing." There is considerable public support for the death squads as the result of perceptions that street children are dangerous criminals. Residents of the poorest communities are often the strongest supporters of violent solutions to local crime, perhaps because their neighborhoods are the least secure.

The most notorious of the death squad killings of street children occurred in 1993 in Rio de Janeiro. At 1 A.M. on July 25th, as 50 homeless youths were sleeping on the grounds of the Candelária Cathedral in the downtown section of the city, a group of gunmen drove up and began shooting (Ellison 1994; Dewees and Klees 1995). Four of the youths died instantly, a fifth was shot and killed as he ran, two more were abducted, beaten, shot and dumped in the gardens of the nearby Museum of Modern Art, and an eighth died several days later, never waking from a coma. Eight others were also shot, but survived their wounds. Three members of the military police were arrested for the crimes, and the shootings were reportedly provoked by an occurrence earlier in the day in which some of the children had allegedly thrown stones at a military police vehicle after one youth had been detained for drug use. The incident captured headlines worldwide. A commission was established to investigate the "Candelária massacre," but its progress was slowed when two of its members were slain in Rio de Janeiro by unidentified gunmen (*Facts on File* 1996). Nevertheless, on April 30, 1996, one of the police officers—Marcos Vinicius Borges Emmanuel, who had admitted to one of the killings—was convicted on six counts of murder, five counts of attempted murder, and several counts of grievous bodily harm, and received a sentence of 309 years (*Facts on File* 1996).[2]

Street children are also the targets of drug gangs. Because Brazil's Protective Child Statute holds that children under 18 years of age may not be arrested unless caught *in the act of* committing a crime, to the drug gangs the youths' impunity makes them ideal couriers. But they are often killed because they know too much, steal too much, or get caught in the cross-fire (Michaels 1993).

The hierarchy of the *favela* drug trade is a vertical one, and children are recruited into the lowest level, serving primarily as lookouts. They progress to running errands for the hillside dealers, and if they are successful, they begin delivering drugs to customers. Survivors from these operations may become armed "controllers" (security guards who protect the operation and proceeds of drug transactions). Finally, there are the corporate levels of the local drug business, but few children ever last that long. Most die while they are still at the lower end of the hierarchy. When a hillside dealer is dissatisfied with a child's work, or decides that the youth is dangerous as a witness, he or she is simply killed (Raphael and Berkman 1992). And altogether, it is estimated that as many as four to five street children are murdered each day throughout Brazil, and two each day in Rio de Janeiro alone (ICRI 1996).

Intervention Strategies

Although there have been many proposals and programs for addressing the problems of Brazilian street youth (Eisenstein 1993, 1994; Kirsch 1995), it would appear that only minimal headway has been achieved. At the most general level, programs appear to be of four types (1) the correctional approach, (2) the rehabilitative perspective, (3) outreach strategies, and (4) the preventive outlook (Lusk 1989).

The *correctional approach* views street children as a matter for juvenile justice organizations. This correctional vision seems to dominate the thinking of much of the public and criminal justice authorities. The result is that thousands of street children are housed in institutions. In Brazil, the National Foundation for Child Welfare (FUNABEM) operates twenty treatment centers and "reform" schools for abandoned and delinquent youth. Conditions in these facilities have been described as both crowded and abusive (Lusk 1989). However, some changes appear to be under-way, involving the substitution of correctional initiatives with community-based treatment alternatives.

The *rehabilitative approach* has been gaining momentum throughout Latin America. This perspective holds that street children are not delinquents as much as they are victims of poverty, child abuse and neglect, and untenable living conditions. Because street children are seen as having been harmed by their environments, hundreds of church and voluntary programs have been organized in their behalf. These typically provide housing, drug detoxification, education, and/or work programs. But there is a difficulty. The programs benefit only a limited number of youths, and are unable to address the needs of the millions of boys and girls who continue to call the streets their home.

Because the institutional capacities and resources of virtually all programs are limited and unable to accommodate the overwhelming majority of street children, services are also provided through a variety of *outreach strategies*. In São Paulo, for example, the Catholic Church supports young lay workers who provide educational, counseling, and advocacy services to children in a street setting. In addition to teaching basic hygiene, literacy, and business skills, the general program approach is to instill self-reliance and empowerment so that children will find solutions to their problems. However, it would appear that this street educator model is overly ideological, and fails to deal with the immediate physical and safety needs of street children. Most recently, outreach strategies have been focusing on HIV prevention and risk reduction (Wiik et al. 1989; Siqueira et al. 1992). The effectiveness of these initiatives, however, is unclear.

The *preventive approach* attempts to address the fundamental and underlying problem of childhood poverty. In this regard, UNICEF is conducting educational campaigns to alert policy makers to the causes of children moving to the streets. In addition to policy advocacy, UNICEF provides technical assistance and support for promising local efforts. Those receiving UNICEF's focused attention are of two types (1) programs that provide daytime activities, schooling, jobs, and other alternatives to street work for high risk children, and (2) efforts focusing on the prevention of family disintegration—cooperative day care centers, family planning clinics, small business services, and community kitchens (Lusk 1989).

The most comprehensive effort on behalf of Brazilian street youth is the National Movement for Street Children (Movimento Nacional de Meninos e Meninas de Rua/MNMMR), a nationwide coalition of street children and adult educators founded in 1985 (Raphael and Berkman 1992). MNMMR initiatives focus on shifting the management of street children away from the criminal justice system, codifying the rights of children into law, and structuring innovative approaches for providing education and training for youths directly on the streets where they live. MNMMR projects are targeting an estimated 80,000 youths, the great majority of whom work on the streets and live in nearby *favelas*, with the remaining actually living on the streets.

Postscript

Street children in Brazilian cities are legion. Their actual numbers are difficult to estimate, however, and have often been exaggerated. As one observer put it:

They seem to be everywhere: begging in front of restaurants, peddling cigarettes in sidewalk cafes, shining shoes outside the train station, washing clothes in public fountains. Take a morning stroll on the elegant, black-and-white mosaic sidewalk that curves along Rio's Copacabana Beach and you'll smell them; dozens sleep under the palms there, and the beach serves as a toilet (Brookes 1991:14).

For those who work the streets during the day, returning to their *favela* homes at night, life is harsh and unkind. For the rest who live in the streets day and night, life is mean and unusually short. And for the great majority of Brazil's street children, it would appear that few changes are likely. Prostitution, drug use, infections, and illiteracy are common, yet there are few programs available to address the many needs of youths.

After his election in 1991, Brazilian President Collor de Mello announced a dramatic plan to build 5,000 model schools called CIACs (Centros Integrados de Apoio à Criança/Integrated support Centers for Children) for indigent children and youth over a four-year period. They were conceived to offer indigent youths comprehensive classroom instruction and after school care, three meals a day, medical and psychological attention, shower facilities, sports and cultural activities, and a library. But by the time President Collor was removed from office on charges of fraud and embezzlement, only twenty had been built, and only a few of these had actually been opened. And not surprisingly, the future of the remaining schools continues to be in doubt. In the meantime, as poverty endures, the numbers of street children slowly increase, as does their involvement in drug use, prostitution, crime, and HIV risk behaviors.

Note

1. See Caracas (Venezuela) *El Universal*, 4 Oct. 1985, pp. 4, 30; Caracas *Zeta*, 12–23 Sept. 1985, pp. 39–46; Manaus (Brazil) *Jornal Do Comercio*, 20 May 1986, p. 16; Bogota *El Tiempo*, 1 June 1986, p. 3A; Medellin *El Colombiano*, 22 July 1986, p. 16-A; Bogota *El Tiempo*, 6 Oct. 1986, p. 7A; Lima (Peru) *El Nacional*, 14 Nov. 1986, p. 13; La Paz (Bolivia) *Presencia*, 3 March 1988, Sec. 2, p. 1; São Paulo (Brazil) *Folha de São Paulo*, 11 June 1987, p. A29; Buenos Aires (Argentina) *La Prensa*, 20 June 1987, p. 9; São Paulo *O Estado de São Paulo*, 8 March 1988, p. 18; Bogota *El Espectador*, 2 April 1988, pp. 1A, 10A; La Paz *El Diario*, 21 Oct. 1988, p. 3; Cochabamba (Bolivia) *Los Tiempos*, 13 June 1989, p. B5; São Paulo *O Estado de São Paulo*, 18 June 1989, p. 32; Rio de Janeiro (Brazil) *Manchete*, 28 Oct. 1989, pp. 20–29; Philadelphia *Inquirer*, 21 Sept. 1986, p. 25A; Timothy Ross, "Bolivian Paste Fuels Basuco Boom," *WorldAIDS*, Sept. 1989, p. 9.

2. Emmanuel's sentence of 309 years was largely symbolic, however, since the maximum legal sentence in Brazil is 30 years (*Facts on File* 1996).

8

Epilogue

HIV/AIDS Harm Reduction Initiatives

"Harm reduction" is a concept that is difficult to define with any degree of precision. Its essential feature, however, is the attempt to ameliorate the adverse health, social, legal, and/or economic consequences associated with the use of mood-altering drugs. As such, harm reduction is neither a policy nor a program, but rather, a principle that suggests that managing drug misuse is more appropriate than attempting to stop it altogether. Within this context, harm reduction, or "harm minimization" as it is also termed in a number of countries, can mean different things to different people, groups, cultures, and nations. Most broadly, it can refer to any variety of policies and policy goals, including

1. *Advocacy for Changes in Drug Policies*—legalization, decriminalization, ending the drug prohibition, reduction of criminal sanctions for drug-related crimes, changes in drug paraphernalia laws.
2. *HIV/AIDS-Related Interventions*—needle/syringe exchange programs, HIV prevention/intervention programs, bleach and condom distribution programs, referrals for HIV and other sexually transmitted disease (STD) testing; referrals for HIV and other STD medical care and management, referrals for HIV/AIDS-related psychological care and case management.
3. *Broader Drug Treatment Options*—methadone maintenance by primary care physicians, changes in methadone regulations, heroin substitution programs, new experimental treatments, treatment on demand.
4. *Drug Abuse Management for Those Who Wish to Continue Using Drugs*—counseling and clinical case management programs that promote safer and more responsible drug use.

5. *Ancillary Interventions*—housing and other entitlements, healing centers, support and advocacy groups (Inciardi and Harrison 1999).

Harm reduction per se is not officially a part of American drug policy, and in fact, the very term "harm reduction" has become so value-laden among many U.S. drug strategists and politicians that it is rarely articulated within government circles. This has occurred, for the most part, because "harm reduction" is often used interchangeably with such expressions as drug legalization and marijuana decriminalization. But advocating harm reduction does not necessarily mean promoting the legalization of heroin, cocaine, and other currently illegal drugs. Rather, it can focus on many different alternatives, including drug abuse education, prevention, and treatment. And curiously in this regard, one of the first and oldest harm reduction initiatives in the world—methadone maintenance—originated in the United States more than three decades ago.

In many parts of the world, the appearance of HIV has led to a widespread intensifying of commitments to harm reduction approaches to drug use. Within this context, the focus of this epilogue is what constitutes harm reduction in Brazil, a review of some of Brazil's experiences with harm reduction, and an examination of some of the issues associated with implementing harm reduction initiatives in developing nations.

Harm Reduction and Injection Drug Use

In Brazil, harm reduction is a relatively new phenomenon. As a result, little has been documented about the scope, experience, or effectiveness of harm reduction strategies. What is clear, however, is that the concept in the Brazilian context is far more narrowly focused than in other parts of the world, and emerged specifically in response to the HIV/AIDS epidemic among injection drug users.

Injection drug use is a primary vector of HIV transmission in Brazil. However, because injection drug users lack political power, live in social isolation, and are discriminated against—even by noninjecting drug users—they are seldomly found in traditional substance abuse treatment settings or health services programs, and are reluctant to participate in either research, demonstration, or public health projects. The lack of attention to injectors, and noninjecting drug users as well, demonstrates that until recently, they were not targeted by HIV prevention initiatives and reflects the widespread social marginalization of the entire drug-using population.

On the whole, Brazilian health officials were slow to implement *any* programs for AIDS prevention. Scarce resources were frequently reserved for vaccination programs and for efforts to combat such tropical diseases as malaria, Chagas' disease (a parasitic infection transmitted by insects), and schistosomiasis (a parasitic disease transmitted through blood flukes), which together affect the health of millions of Brazilians (Flowers 1988; Brazilian Ministry of Health 1997b). In fact, during the mid-1980s the Brazilian National Secretary of Health declared that AIDS prevention research would not be a priority, for as long as it was restricted to "minority" groups. The Secretary of Health justified this decision with the argument that Brazil had other, more serious, endemic diseases that resulted from the abject poverty of much of the general population (Lima et al. 1992). Reacting to the stigmatization of "minority group" labeling, the gay community mobilized to form advocacy groups, and as a result, during the late 1980s and early 1990s most prevention programs were organized by and directed toward men who have sex with men.

For the general public in Brazil, government-sponsored education and information campaigns first appeared during the second half of the 1980s (Parker 1992). In early 1987, for example, the government launched a series of television announcements that provided AIDS prevention information for a national audience. These were short-lived, however, because of federal budget cuts and pressure from the Catholic Church (Flowers 1988). Most of the campaigns were designed for a relatively general audience and presented basic information on AIDS risk behaviors. Explicit and controversial messages or promotions targeting specific groups, on the other hand, to a large extent have been absent (Parker 1992). In addition, initial reports in the Brazilian press widely publicized rumors that people with AIDS were deliberately spreading the disease through sexual binges or purposely injecting fellow addicts with contaminated syringes (Flowers 1988). As a result, during the early years of the epidemic little accurate knowledge about HIV reached the public.

Going further, there has been considerable debate in Brazil about the most appropriate and effective mechanisms for developing and targeting materials for diverse audiences. Moreover, groups ranging from gay liberation organizations to conservative sectors of the Catholic Church managed to exert considerable influence on the development of government-sponsored educational campaigns. And finally, many of the obstacles that limited the federal government's ability to design and implement AIDS prevention initiatives have also impacted state and local efforts. When combined with the severe limitations of most state and municipal financial resources, it is not surprising that little in the way of government-sponsored AIDS education and health promotion has emerged in most parts of Brazil (Parker 1992).

By contrast, nongovernmental organizations (NGOs) have played an important role in AIDS education and prevention in Brazil. In late 1985, for example, an association known as *Grupo de Apoio para a Prevenção da AIDS* (Support Group for the Prevention of AIDS) was founded in São Paulo, and became the first volunteer organization in Brazil concerned exclusively with AIDS-related issues. Better known as GAPA, its members were initially comprised of health care workers involved in the treatment of AIDS patients and activists who had previously been involved in gay rights groups. GAPA was the first NGO to become involved in AIDS health promotion, and focused primarily on the instruction of safe sexual practices (Parker 1992).

Shortly after the formation of GAPA, intellectuals and activists in Rio de Janeiro formed *Associação Brasileira Interdisciplinar de AIDS* (ABIA), the Brazilian Interdisciplinary AIDS Association, which developed into a well-respected professional organization and has played an important role as a critic of government policy on AIDS and as a principal designer of health promotion materials. ABIA has been credited with the development of highly focused health promotion materials targeted to diverse populations within Brazil and with supplying many of these items to AIDS service organizations. Less vulnerable to criticism than government produced materials, the AIDS education media developed by ABIA have been among the most direct and explicit available anywhere in Brazil (Parker 1992). Some of ABIA's particularly important campaigns have targeted street children, construction workers, sailors, and gay-identified men. Male, female, and transvestite prostitutes have also been the focus of several campaigns, including an AIDS prevention initiative linked with the Institute for Religious Studies in Rio de Janeiro. Others at significant risk for HIV infection, however, especially injection drug users, were largely overlooked by these efforts. Despite statistical evidence of alarming HIV seroprevalence rates among drug injectors, by the end of the first decade of the epidemic there was still no official policy or programs directed to this particular group (Lima et al. 1992). Even by late 1996, respected Brazilian drug researchers were still lamenting the lack of political attention paid to the public health problems associated with drug abuse in Brazil (Laranjeira and Pinsky 1996).

Syringe Exchange

It was not until 1992 that a harm reduction approach for injection drug users was first discussed by the Brazilian National Program on STD/AIDS. The dialogue revolved around syringe exchange, and with the exception of one pioneering exchange program in Santos, initiated in 1989 but quickly closed under pressure from the Federal Narcotics Council

(Alexandrino 1991), this discussion represented the first government initiative to systematically address the negative consequences of drug use among Brazilians.

The lack of harm reduction strategies for injection drug users in Brazil can be traced to the rigid drug legislation currently in force. Although Brazilian statutes permit the purchase and possession of syringes/needles, current drug laws are tough and anachronistic, which makes such prevention strategies as syringe/needle exchange programs difficult to implement (Barbosa de Carvalho et al. 1996). Brazil's initial antidrug law, passed in 1971, was essentially punitive in nature: it penalized both users and dealers, and ordered hospital treatment for those with chemical dependency. The 1976 law, still in effect, revised and expanded the original statute, as follows:

Article 12   Importing or exporting, shipping, preparing, producing, manufacturing, acquiring, selling, offering for sale, supplying even freely, storing, transporting, carrying with you, keeping, prescribing, administering or delivering in any manner, narcotic substances or those which create physical or psychological dependence, without authorization or accordance with legal regulations:

Penalty   Confinement, from three to fifteen years, and payment of 50 to 360 days-fine.[1]

Article 16   Acquiring, keeping, or carrying, for your own personal use, narcotic substances or those which create physical or psychological dependence, without authorization or accordance with legal regulations:

Penalty   Confinement, from six months to two years, and payment of 20 to 50 days-fine.

According to a number of legal scholars, this language does not necessarily define drug use per se as a crime, but rather, as in the United States, the statutes prohibit possession, manufacture, sale, and distribution (Brazilian Ministry of Health 1991). However, the ambiguity of the legal language serves to exacerbate the debate, and as such many scholars and legislators argue for the creation of a legal document that explicitly decriminalizes drug use or dependency per se, for the purpose of differentiating users from producers, traffickers, and dealers in the eyes of the law. Going further, in the absence of specific paraphernalia restrictions in antidrug laws, the main barrier to the implementation of needle/syringe exchange programs is the language in paragraph two of Article 12, which classifies "instigating, inducing, and/or assisting" the use of drugs as criminal acts, each carrying three- to fifteen-year prison sentences. Because city councils and local governments must comply with federal regulations in this area, HIV/AIDS prevention programs for injection drug users have been impeded by the threat of legal action.

More recently, there has been discussion of harm reduction strategies at the national level sparked by those seeking to reform Brazilian drug laws. Central to these reforms is the legal status of needle/syringe exchange programs, which are key features of harm reduction in Brazil. Among the issues raised in this regard was the recommendation of the 1993 Conference of Ibero-American Health Ministers that experimental interventions (needle/syringe exchange, bleach distribution) be developed to address the grave public health issue of HIV/AIDS. Building on this endorsement of harm reduction strategies, the Brazilian Federal Narcotics Council approved a six-site pilot needle/syringe exchange program proposed by the Ministry of Health in 1994 (*Jornal do Brasil* 1994). Citing the need to make drug use as safe as possible for both individuals and society, the council sanctioned the operation of exchange programs in six Brazilian cities having high HIV incidence and relatively large communities of injection drug users: São Paulo, Belo Horizonte, Santos, Salvador, Rio de Janeiro, and Campo Grande. In part, these cities were also selected because they possessed a relatively well-developed structure for administering the programs, and the council insisted on tight control by their respective municipal health centers. In fact, the council specified that the following guidelines be observed: the project must be highly localized and directed to a specific clientele; there must be oversight, control, and evaluation of the project at every level; and the experimental nature of the project should be emphasized. Importantly, the council also mandated that at least 50 percent of each project's operating budget be applied to drug-use prevention efforts (Federal Narcotics Council 1994).

Organizations at the state level with an interest in HIV/AIDS prevention strategies were quick to act on the favorable decision of the Federal Narcotics Council. Citing a study of 13 cities conducted by the World Health Organization (which included Rio de Janeiro and Santos, Brazil), the São Paulo State Council on AIDS Issues declared harm reduction strategies to be the most effective in controlling the spread of HIV/AIDS among injection drug users (State Council on AIDS Issues 1994). Going further, in 1995 the STD/AIDS Division of the São Paulo State Secretary of Health openly declared its position on harm reduction and delineated appropriate goals and strategies of this approach:

> the harm reduction approach [should] be the primary strategy for the state public health network when working with injection drug users. Although a broader range of actions is necessary when dealing with the issue of drugs,

such as the prevention of use and treatment for substance abusers, the harm reduction strategy without a doubt presents the greatest possibility for short-term impact. The harm reduction strategy asserts that if the rehabilitation of injection drug users demands a great investment and may not be effective in the short-term, it is necessary to adopt methods low in both material and human costs which can quickly produce an impact on HIV prevention in this group. This strategy includes disinfecting injection equipment with bleach, and needle/syringe exchange by injecting drug users. The availability of sterile needles/syringes for injection drug users would diminish the risk not only of HIV infection, but other blood borne infections such as hepatitis, Chagas disease, etc. (State Secretary of Health STD/AIDS Division 1995).

Although their support for needle/syringe exchange was evident, the Secretary of Health clearly asserted that these programs must be linked with broader prevention strategies, such as substance abuse counseling and treatment, in order to achieve the primary goals of harm reduction: prevention of needle/syringe sharing, reduction in the rate of HIV infection among injection drug users, changes in the route of drug administration from injection to noninjection, overall reduction in the use of drugs, and elimination of the use of drugs (State Secretary of Health STD/AIDS Division 1995). Within this context, the Secretary of Health recommended that services offered to injection drug users in any context always include counseling on STD/HIV transmission, needle/syringe cleaning, and condom use. It was further suggested that health service providers that serve large numbers of injection drug users be evaluated for the feasibility of initiating needle/syringe exchange programs as well as bleach and condom distribution initiatives.

Despite the broad-based support for needle exchange efforts demonstrated by both federal and state agencies, the implementation of such projects has been slow and difficult. The Brazilian Ministry of Health piloted two needle/syringe exchange programs in Santos and Salvador in 1995. In Salvador at the Federal University of Bahia, a small prevention program, including needle/syringe exchange, has been operating since March 1995. It provides services to injection drug users, which were practically nonexistent before this, and provides disposable injection equipment, condoms, HIV prevention information, and referrals for medical and social services. Little information is available to international researchers regarding the effectiveness of the program in Salvador, but the fact that it has operated continuously for more than four years speaks to its success. Going further, a report by the investigators in 1997 indicated that more than 5,000 syringes had been exchanged at the four sites since distribution began.

The needle exchange program in Santos was not as fortunate. Shortly after its initiation, it was closed as a result of police action. The Narcotics Police of Santos seized all of the materials used by the Institute for AIDS Research and Study (IEPAS) for this HIV prevention project including 371 eyeglass cases (where the kits containing disposable injection equipment are stored), 500 alcohol swabs for disinfecting the skin, 500 bottles of bleach for disinfecting needles/syringes, and 600 condoms (*O Estado de São Paulo* 1995). The project was later moved to the neighboring area of São Vicente due to the more relaxed political climate and syringe distribution was reinitiated. More recently, the Ministry of Health and the Federal Narcotics Council of the Ministry of Justice gave joint approval for seven needle/syringe exchange programs to be funded by international institutions (*O Estado de São Paulo* 1996b).

Before this decision, needle/syringe exchange programs had *never* existed in Rio de Janeiro. Although Rio de Janeiro has the second largest number of reported AIDS cases in Brazil, it had reported fewer than 900 cases among injection drug users through March 1997, ranking it far below other cities in cases among this population (Brazilian Ministry of Health 1997a; State Secretary of Health STD/AIDS Division 1997). Perhaps as a result of this trend few studies of this population have been conducted. Those that have dealt with injection drug users in Rio de Janeiro typically were small-scale epidemiologic or seroprevalence studies that did not provide any intervention component (see Telles et al. 1994). However, one harm reduction project is underway in Rio de Janeiro and has succeeded in accessing injection drug users (Telles et al. 1998; Telles 1999). Due to the legal issues surrounding needle/syringe exchange and communications from the federal police denouncing such activities, however, the distribution of needles/syringes has been intermittant (Telles 1997, 1999).

Other Harm Reduction Initiatives

In the United States, as noted earlier in this discussion, harm reduction is considered to encompass such activities as HIV/AIDS interventions, drug treatment, drug substitution therapy (maintenance on drug of choice from legal source), safer and more responsible drug use, reductions in penalties for drug-related crimes, changes in paraphernalia laws, and decriminalization/legalization of controlled substances. In Brazil, on the other hand, it occupies a narrow definition that typically includes needle/syringe exchange, bleach disinfection, substitution of noninjection drug use for injection use, traditional drug treatment, and general HIV/AIDS prevention education.

Other aspects of harm reduction that have extreme visibility in different parts of the world receive little attention in Brazil. Efforts to modify the existing drug statutes have encountered virtually unlimited resistance from authorities and experts in the field. Sparked by Rio de Janeiro Governor Marcello Alencar's declaration to "smoke one and see how it is," the decriminalization of marijuana was among the suggested proposals to be debated by the Congress in February of 1996 (*O Estado de São Paulo* 1996a). The legislation brought by a congressman from Minas Gerais proposed that the existing laws be modified to distinguish between drug users and traffickers, and to differentiate between "hard" and "soft" drugs. Brazilian criminalist Arthur Lavigne was among those who criticized this proposal:

> This new law will not punish the man who buys drugs because he is a user, but will give a penalty of at least 10 years in prison to those who sell drugs, who may do so out of absolute [financial] necessity; well, you should send everyone to jail or no one (*O Estado de São Paulo* 1996a).

Former Rio de Janeiro Mayor Cesar Maia also supported drug prohibition and said of the proposal:

> I'm absolutely opposed to legalization, even of "soft" drugs." According to the mayor, legalizing drug use was an experience that didn't work in any of the countries that tried it. "The results were catastrophic; today, no one talks about drug legalization anymore (*O Estado de São Paulo* 1996a).

Perhaps not surprisingly, the proposed changes to existing drug legislation have not been enacted.

Other *legal* dimensions of the harm reduction movement are somewhat irrelevant in the Brazilian context. Paraphernalia laws are nonexistent and needles/syringes are generally not used as evidence of law violations. Indeed, syringes/needles can be purchased in pharmacies without a prescription, at relatively low prices. However, anecdotal reports in focus groups with injection drug users suggest that people who "look like drug users" or fit a popular stereotype of a drug user may have problems purchasing injection equipment in pharmacies or may be asked to pay "special" prices. Injectors also indicated that it is difficult to obtain needles after regular business hours, as only "emergency" drug stores are open on nights and weekends, and they are generally located at great distances from low-income neighborhoods. As such, the issue of sterile injection paraphernalia for injectors in Brazil revolves not around legality or availability, but accessibility.

In the absence of paraphernalia restrictions, needle/syringe exchange programs have been hampered by the legislation that classifies "instigating, inducing, and/or assisting" the use of drugs as criminal acts. In a recent effort to modify this statute, which is frequently interpreted by authorities to encompass needle/syringe exchange, a bill was introduced to the Congress that would add the following language to the existing law: "with the exception of actions undertaken by the public health authority" (Silva 1997). While this bill was under study, the State of São Paulo took things one step further in September 1997 by passing a new law authorizing the State Secretary of Health to exchange syringes for drug users (Diário Oficial 1997). São Paulo is the first state to have such a law, but plans to begin implementation of the new statute slowly in order to avoid public resistance (Segatto 1997). In fact, according to Pedro Chequer, the Coordinator of the National AIDS Prevention Program, several agencies have *discretely* implemented syringe exchange in the hope of avoiding opposition, but he placed the number of programs at fewer than ten nationally (Segatto 1997).

Accessibility to other harm reduction strategies is also a problem in Brazil. Drug abuse treatment is frequently restricted to a few religious institutions without the resources to meet the demand, and to private clinics, which are expensive and therefore not accessible to the majority of injection drug users (Barbosa de Carvalho et al. 1996). In fact, it was not until December 1996 that the first public free-of-charge, residential, drug treatment clinic was opened in São Paulo state, which is the most economically progressive region of Brazil (Tomaleza 1996). Going further, condom distribution programs directed to drug users are uncommon, especially when compared to those operating for male and female sex workers, the gay community, and sex partners of HIV-infected persons. Consequently, rates of condom use among this population are extremely low, with one study reporting that 90.2 percent and 91.3 percent of drug-using men and women, respectively, did not use condoms all or most of the time (Inciardi et al. 1996).

As described earlier in Chapter 5, an effort was made by the authors to introduce the female condom to drug using men and women in Rio de Janeiro, and interviews suggested that participants found the female condom to be an acceptable method of HIV risk reduction (Surratt et al. 1998). However, given Brazil's economic turmoil, high rates of indigency and other social problems, conflicts between state and federal jurisdictions, and the opposition of the Catholic Church to broad-based condom distribution, the future of the female condom remains uncertain, as does the future of other neophyte harm reduction initiatives.

The HIV prevention/intervention program initiated in Rio de Janeiro by the authors of this monograph, which lasted from 1994 through 1998, still stands as the only large-scale AIDS prevention effort aimed at drug-using *favela* residents. The project had an impact, and even more than a year after the project's closing, former clients were returning to the research offices seeking help.

Postscript

Harm reduction strategies have demonstrated numerous achievements in increasing the quality of life for drug-involved populations around the world. Many harm reduction advocates, however, tend to have an "all or nothing" philosophy, denigrating both the efforts and the accomplishments of those who do not share their zeal. This difficulty was faced by the authors during the 1998 International Conference on Drug Related Harm in São Paulo, Brazil (Inciardi et al. 1998). Because needle exchange had not been included as a component of the Rio de Janeiro–based HIV/AIDS intervention program described in Chapters 3 and 4, the authors were ridiculed by a number of harm reduction advocates from the United States. The project was denounced as "tantamount to genocide" and a reflection of "the failed U.S. AIDS policy." In response to such critiques, it must be emphasized that syringe exchange programs are important, and Brazil is moving in the right direction in this regard. But at the same time, focusing all of one's efforts and ideological stamina solely on syringe exchange tends to be somewhat anachronistic—particularly when a large portion of the drug-using population is comprised of noninjectors. In the Rio de Janeiro project, for example, more than 90 percent of the drug-using clients were noninjectors. Almost 9 percent tested positive for HIV infection—an extremely high rate for a noninjecting population. Moreover, injection drug users are exposed to HIV infection through sexual contact—an important issue in Brazil given the fact that the heterosexual spread of HIV and AIDS are increasing.

The project in Rio de Janeiro was an appropriate first step. When it was fielded in 1994, there were no needle exchange programs anywhere in Brazil, and there were no community-based intervention programs targeting indigent or even low-income drug users. Among the more than 1,600 clients that were eventually recruited, almost 70 percent had never received any HIV/AIDS prevention information—pamphlets, condoms, bleach, referral sources, or anything else. Needle exchange programs become feasible only in conjunction with these "first generation" education and prevention efforts.

In the years since the initiation of the authors' AIDS prevention project in Rio de Janeiro, the harm reduction movement in Brazil has gained considerable momentum. For example,

- Between 1993 and 1997, 559 projects were funded by Brazil's National STD/AIDS Program in the areas of education, behavioral change, and communications activities.
- In 1996, the National STD/AIDS Program initiated the National Brazilian Prevention Conference, a countrywide forum for the

discussion of methods appropriate for health education and prevention.

- In 1997, the Brazilian government launched a sentinal project in STD clinics and hospital emergency rooms to monitor national rates of HIV infection.
- In 1998, Brazil negotiated a loan agreement with the World Bank to fund AIDS-II, a large scale program for the prevention, diagnosis, and treatment of HIV/AIDS.
- And in 1999, the Brazilian government distributed 2 million female condoms and 200 million male condoms, and installed 133 free AIDS testing units nationwide.

Note

1. Because Brazilian currency tends to change and/or lose its value rapidly, income is frequently calculated in terms of the number of minimum salaries earned, rather than a fixed monetary value. Thus, "50 to 360 days-fine" refers to the wages that would be earned during this time period.

Appendix A
The NIDA Standard Intervention

The HIV/AIDS intervention program presented here includes a number of specific steps, each of which is described at length in the pages that follow. These procedures may be followed by public health workers and counselors who met with their clients in office settings. An important point for anyone conducting this intervention is to use language that the clients will be comfortable with.

Session I: HIV Prevention Counseling

Provide your client a comfortable place to sit in a private setting, and introduce yourself by name and role as a health educator/interventionist. Summarize what you are going to talk about and why. Although a large portion of the material to be covered seems didactic in nature, remember to pace the session to allow questions and interaction. By asking and encouraging questions, listening for concerns, and offering support, you can personalize this session for each of your clients. Use language appropriate for the educational level of the client.

Session I should include:

- a discussion of HIV prevention material listed on the attached set of 15 A cue cards;
- a rehearsal of how to use condoms;
- a rehearsal of how to clean injection equipment;
- the distribution of hygiene products (condoms, bleach, water, alcohol swabs, and Band-Aids);
- a discussion of the HIV test; and
- the distribution of HIV-related literature.

The A Cue Cards

In brief, the 15 A cue cards provide the following talking points:

1. basic information about HIV/AIDS disease;
2. truths and myths about how someone gets infected;
3. behaviors that put people at risk;
4. how and why to use condoms;
5. how and why to clean injection equipment;

6. risks related to cocaine;
7. the benefits of drug treatment;
8. the meaning of the HIV test; and,
9. healthy behaviors to practice if infected.

The cue cards should be presented as follows:

HIV Disease
Cue Card A.1 provides basic information about AIDS and its viral source.

Course of HIV Infection
Cue Card A.2 shows the usual course of HIV Infection and AIDS, beginning with first becoming infected and ending with death.

Transmission Routes
Cue Card A.3 prompts you to outline the various ways HIV is transmitted (semen, blood, and through pregnancy) and Card A.3 also denounces myths about HIV transmission (such as by casual contact, saliva, tears, toilet seats, and insect bites).

Risky Behaviors
Cue Card A.4 prompts you to describe behaviors that put people at risk. Ask the client to assess his or her own risk situation as you discuss this card. Emphasize the risks associated with the common practice of sharing drug paraphernalia (needles, syringes, cookers, cotton, rinse water). Cue Card A.5 describes the risks of indirect sharing. Explain how using a "donor" syringe also presents significant transmission risks.

Also emphasize the risks of unprotected sex, especially with persons who have a history of drug use or multiple sexual partners. Warn against the disinhibiting effects of drugs and alcohol that may lead to risky behavior or even jeopardize the immune system. Discuss the common risk factors for HIV and other sexually transmitted diseases, and the effect of these diseases on HIV transmission.

Risks Associated with Crack or Cocaine
Cue Card A.6 prompts you to point out the risks related to cocaine. Emphasize especially the link between using cocaine and crack, and losing the ability to practice safer sex, and also how the drugs may compromise the immune system. Tell clients that one way to reduce their risk is to stop using drugs. If they believe they cannot, urge them to at least avoid injecting drugs and to practice safer sex.

Crack cocaine has become a leading drug of choice among many drug users. Trading or bartering or exchanging sex for money, crack, or other drugs is on the increase with greater risk for HIV among heavier users. Many of the people at risk are women. Therefore, there is a seriously deadly relationship between drugs and sex.

Rehearsal of Condom Use

Cue Card A.7 asks "Why Use Condoms?" Review the benefits of condoms to prevent the spread of AIDS (and other sexually transmitted diseases, which in turn can promote the transmission of HIV). *At this point, stop your presentation and offer an unopened condom to the client.* Open the package carefully and advise how to avoid tearing the product as you do so. Explain that the tip of the condom should be pinched to release the air and allow room for the ejaculate. Unroll the condom over a penis model, explaining that condoms are never to be pulled on. *This demonstration should be done at least once for every client.*

When demonstrating condom use, explain that to be effective, the condom must be worn before penetration and all the way through sex; it must also be positioned all the way down on the shaft of the penis.

Explain that after orgasm, one partner should hold on to the condom at its base to keep it from slipping off. Talk about the correct removal and disposal of the condom after use. Ask the client to demonstrate his or her proficiency by fitting a condom on the model. Continue such playback until proficiency is achieved.

Discuss the types of condoms that protect against HIV transmission and the types of lubricants that can be safely used with condoms. Briefly introduce the *female condom,* using Cue Card A.8.

The Female Condom

Explain that the female condom has several advantages over the male condom, both as a contraceptive and as a sexually transmitted disease prevention method. First, it is primarily woman-controlled. With the female condom, women are not as dependent on the cooperation of sex partners to protect themselves from HIV and other sexually transmitted diseases. Second, the female condom is inserted before intercourse, providing additional protection against infections from pre-ejaculated fluids. Third, the female condom protects a greater proportion of the vagina, which also provides further protection against sexually transmitted diseases. Fourth, the female condom has less risk of rupture than the male condom. Other advantages are that it causes less loss of sensitivity (because of its loose fit), it permits penetration before complete erection of the penis, and it permits continued intimacy in the resolution phase of intercourse since it need not be removed immediately.

You can also explain that tests have shown that the female condom has a lower leakage rate than the male condom, and that it has been found to be as effective as other barrier methods at preventing conception. Furthermore, in simulated laboratory testing of the female condom, there was no viral leakage for HIV.

Stopping Unsafe Sex Practices

Clearly, condoms are not the only way to reduce the risk of infection through sexual behavior. To personalize the session, offer a flexible array of risk reduction practices, such as

- point out that one of the ways to reduce risk is not to have sex;
- also, there is nonpenetrative sex and mutual masturbation;

- one can always reduce the number of sex partners, particularly those who inject drugs or who have many partners of their own; you can add that even reducing the number of partners from five to three can reduce risk somewhat;
- finally, *emphasize that one of the best ways to reduce risk is to use condoms with all partners.*

How to Talk with Your Partner about Safer Sex

Cue Card A.9 offers some suggestions on talking about safer sex. Since this kind of communication may be difficult for many clients, stress that having unprotected sex with a person infected with HIV is one of the main ways of contracting this disease; therefore, your life may depend on your ability to discuss practicing safer sex.

Lead into a discussion of the points on the card by explaining the following to the client:

Talking to your partner(s) about practicing safer sex is an important first step in the process of protecting yourself from HIV. However, it may not be easy to talk to your partner(s) about having safer sex. Just the thought of bringing this issue up with your partner(s) may make you feel uncomfortable or embarrassed or you may worry about how your partner(s) will react. These are all normal concerns that we all share.

In order to make it easier to talk to your partner(s) about practicing safer sex, you must first make a firm decision and commitment to yourself that the only kind of sex you will have is protected sex. This will make it easier to stand firm if your partner tries to convince you that you don't need to use protection with him/her.

Discuss the points on the card. When you have finished, emphasize again the importance of talking about safer sex. Remind the client that HIV is a fact of life: not talking about it will not make it go away, and talking about it and practicing safer sex may save your life.

Needle and Syringe Cleaning and Disinfection Guidelines

Much remains to be learned before practical disinfection guidelines for injection drug users can be established. Until then, recommendations for cleaning and disinfecting procedures are likely to abound. Such techniques should be promoted as a means of reducing but not eliminating the risk of HIV transmission. Clearly, it is preferable for injectors to not share and always use sterile supplies. When this is not possible, cleaning and disinfection techniques should be considered.

It is important for clients to attempt to disinfect all injection equipment that is known or suspected to have been used by someone else. It is also important for clients to be aware of risks from indirect sharing practices.

Full-strength bleach is one of the more effective disinfectants. If bleach is not available, a mixture of detergent and water, alcohol, or even vinegar may be used in an attempt to clean injection equipment as thoroughly as possible. This may not offer 100 percent protection, but it is likely to reduce the risk of contaminated supplies spreading infection.

Cleaning and disinfecting are best accomplished immediately after injection equipment has been used, before residual blood begins to clot and dry up. Studies suggest that an effective bleach disinfection procedure requires all contaminated surfaces to be exposed twice to full-strength bleach for at least 30 seconds. Also, remind clients to use *new* bleach. (Bleach begins to lose its strength after it has been open for a while.)

Rehearsal of Needle and Syringe Cleaning

Cue Card A.10 asks "Why Clean Needles and Syringes?" Review the health risks associated with using drugs and, especially, sharing all equipment, cookers, cotton, and rinse water. When clients believe that they cannot stop drug use or equipment sharing, tell them that needle cleaning is imperative and repeat the importance of avoiding indirect sharing. Stop your presentation and demonstrate how to use water and bleach to clean injection equipment. *This demonstration should be done at least once with every client.*

The following needle and syringe cleaning materials should be available:

- cup with rinse water;
- container with full-strength, household bleach; and
- empty cup.

Stress that only NEW, full-strength, household bleach and clean, never-used water should be used for bleach disinfection of needles and syringes.

Draw full-strength bleach through the submerged needle to fill the barrel of the syringe. Shake and/or tap the barrel with your finger to agitate the contents for 30 seconds. Squirt out the bleach to dispose of it, or discharge it into the cooker if this is also being cleaned. **REPEAT this a second time.**

After using the bleach, rinse the syringe and needle. Draw clean water through the submerged needle to fill the syringe and squirt out to dispose of it. **REPEAT.** If the cooker is also being cleaned, water can be used to flush out the residual bleach. **DO NOT REUSE WATER OR BLEACH.**

Emphasize that all injection equipment should be cleaned after each use. Make sure to add that **CLEANING WATER/BLEACH SHOULD ALWAYS BE DISCARDED INTO A SINK, TOILET, SEWER, OR DISCARD BOTTLE. IT IS HAZARDOUS WASTE.**

NOTE: Suggest that clients take the syringe apart (remove the plunger) to improve the cleaning/disinfection of parts that might not be reached by flushing with water and bleach.

Ask the client to demonstrate his or her proficiency by cleaning the needle and syringe as directed. Continue such playback until proficiency is achieved.

Stopping Unsafe Drug Use

Cleaning needles is not the only way to reduce the risks associated with using drugs. To personalize the session, offer several possible ways to control unsafe drug use. Point out to your client that:

- One way to reduce risk is to stop using drugs, or at least reducing the frequency of use.
- If they continue to use drugs, they should stop sharing, borrowing, lending, or renting equipment—including indirect sharing.

Review cleaning points using Cue Card A.11.

Emphasize that while stopping these behaviors is best, reducing their frequency will give the client a greater degree of protection against AIDS than he or she has now.

Benefits of Drug Treatment

Cue Card A.12 prompts you to highlight the benefits of drug treatment—to get off drugs, to provide social support for coping with AIDS or kicking the habit, and to connect clients with health and social services. Mention the opportunity to connect with other people like themselves, too.

HIV Antibody Testing

Cue Card A.13 prompts you to review the HIV antibody testing procedure and the meaning of HIV antibody test results, including the uncertain nature of negative test results and the uncertain prognosis of positive results. Discuss both the advantages and disadvantages of testing, and pay special attention to early medical treatment and confidentiality issues.

Infection

Cue Card A.14 prompts you to outline healthy behaviors for a client to practice if infected. Encourage early medical intervention, and explain the dangers of taking in more virus by unsafe practices. Stress that practicing safer sex is important even if you are infected. Review ways for your clients to take good care of their health.

Partner Notification

Cue Card A.15 prompts you to address partner notification issues. Partners may want to consider changing their behaviors and may want to seek HIV testing.

Literature, Referrals, and Hygiene Kit

Before wrapping up the session, probe for questions and provide written material about the information discussed in the cue card session. In addition to factual information about HIV disease, HIV transmission, and risk reduction, the literature should include a local referral list to drug treatment agencies (if available) and a local referral list for other HIV prevention and testing agencies. In addition, give all clients a hygiene kit.

HIV Testing

For those subjects who are willing, blood should be drawn for HIV testing on the same day as Session I (immediately following, if possible). Before drawing blood, explain (1) any foreseeable discomfort, (2) the expected benefits of testing, (3) the extent to which records will be held confidential, and (4) that the blood test is voluntary.

Session II: HIV Booster Counseling

Session II provides HIV posttest counseling to people who have been tested, and a risk reduction booster session to all clients whether or not they have been tested. The intervention should include two sets of counseling materials for clients who (1) are not tested (the sero-unaware group) or who test negative for the virus (the seronegative group), and (2) test positive for the virus.

Session II should be conducted in a private, one-on-one interview format. The expected duration is 20 to 40 minutes, but may be longer for seropositive clients.

Seronegative and Sero-Unaware Clients

The content of Session II will be the same for clients who test negative for the virus and for those who are sero-unaware. The content will include

- provision of the test result, if applicable;
- a discussion of risk reduction and the meaning of HIV positive and negative test results, based on the attached set of two B cue cards;
- a review of HIV prevention, using Cue Cards A.3 through A.12); and
- distribution of literature about HIV and HIV referral.

Provision of Test Results

When applicable, inform the client of the result of the HIV test result and show the lab slip. Allow time for the client to react and to verbalize feelings.

HIV Test Results Cue Cards

Explain what negative *and* positive results mean and how clients can reduce the spread of HIV. In brief, the B cue cards provide the following talking points: (1) seronegative results mean that HIV antibodies have not been detected but can show up later, (2) seropositive results mean that a client (and possibly friends and sexual partners with whom risk behaviors have been practiced) is infected and can infect others.

HIV Prevention Cue Cards

Review the material from Session I on HIV prevention using Cue Cards A.2 through A.12.

Distribution of Literature, Hygiene Kit, and Referrals

Provide written literature about the information discussed in the cue card session. In addition to factual information about HIV disease, HIV transmission, and risk reduction, the literature should include a local referral list to drug treatment agencies (if available) and a local referral list for other HIV prevention and testing agencies. In addition, give all clients a hygiene kit.

Seropositive Clients

The content of Session II for clients who test positive for the virus should include

- provision of the test result;
- a discussion of the meaning of HIV positive test result, based on the attached set of three C cue cards;
- a discussion of medical follow-up and early treatment; and
- the distribution of literature about HIV and HIV referrals.

Provision of Test Results

Seropositive test results should always be given by trained counselors. When giving a client a positive result, show the lab slip. Allow time for the client to react and to verbalize feelings.

Some crisis intervention may be needed when a client has been informed that he or she is seropositive. A helpful response should include empathy, warmth, a positive regard for the client and his or her feelings, and an effort to help the client understand the situation and options clearly. Your specific goals should be to

- listen actively and with concern;
- encourage open expression of feelings (unless the client is out of control);
- help the client to understand the crisis;
- help the client to gradually accept reality;
- encourage the client to explore new ways of coping with problems;
- link the client to a support network; and
- reinforce newly learned coping devices and follow up after the immediate crisis is resolved.

HIV Test Results Cue Cards

Explain what positive results mean and what actions should be taken next. In brief, the three C cue cards provide the following talking points:

- seropositive results mean that a client (and possibly friends or sexual partners with whom risk behaviors have been practiced) is infected;

- healthy behaviors to practice if infected with HIV;
- partner notification issues; and,
- ways to prevent spreading HIV to others.

Medical Treatment Advice

Inform all clients that it is important for seropositive individuals to seek medical care. They should have blood testing done to determine how the immune system is functioning, and discuss with their doctor early treatments that may prevent infections and slow the progression of HIV disease. Discuss approved medical treatments that are locally available that can help avert symptoms and opportunistic infections.

Emphasize the importance of staying in a medical treatment program, of getting regular checkups, and of learning about new medical procedures. Note that infected people can probably stay healthier by reducing drug use; getting good nutrition, sleep, and exercise; and by cultivating a positive attitude (with support groups and counseling).

Distribution of Literature, HIV Referrals, and Hygiene Kit

Provide written literature about the information discussed in the cue card session. In addition to factual information about the meaning of test results (a copy of Cue Card C.1), healthy behaviors (a copy of Cue Card C.2) and local partner notification laws, the literature should include

- a local referral list to medical treatment agencies, clinics, and physicians in the area who treat HIV/AIDS (if available); and
- a local referral list of drug treatment agencies (if available).

In addition, give all clients a hygiene kit.

A.1

What is AIDS?

- AIDS stands for acquired immune deficiency syndrome. This disease is a serious health problem in our country and around the world.

- National and Local Statistics.

- AIDS is caused by the human immunodeficiency virus, commonly known as HIV.

- HIV can destroy the body's ability to fight off infections and disease.

A.2

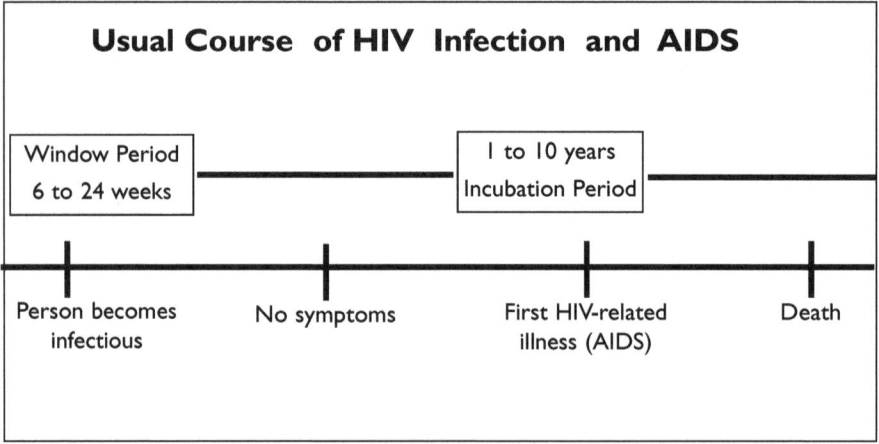

Usual Course of HIV Infection and AIDS

Window Period
6 to 24 weeks

1 to 10 years
Incubation Period

Person becomes
infectious

No symptoms

First HIV-related
illness (AIDS)

Death

A.3

How Does Someone Get Infected?

- HIV, the AIDS virus, is present in semen, blood, and vaginal fluid.

- HIV is transmitted
  —by sexual acts like oral, anal, and vaginal intercourse,
  —by sharing needles and other drug injection equipment, or
  —by receiving blood from an infected person.

- HIV is transmitted from mother to child during pregnancy or the birth process. It is possibly also transmitted by breast-feeding.

- You *can't* get HIV through everyday contact such as shaking hands or hugging.

- You *can't* get HIV from saliva, sweat, tears, urine, or feces.

- You *can't* get HIV from clothes, a telephone, or a toilet seat.

- You *can't* get HIV from a dry kiss.

- You *can't* get HIV from a mosquito bite or other insect bites.

A.4

What Behavior Puts You at Risk

- Sharing needles and syringes.

- Sharing cookers, cotton, and rinse water.

- Not using a condom or barrier during vaginal, oral, or anal sex.

- You increase your chances or getting HIV if you have unprotected sex with
  —someone who has several sex partners; or
  —someone who injects drugs.

- Using alcohol or other drugs can be risky because
  —alcohol and drugs may increase your desire to have sex and make you less careful;
  —alcohol and drugs may weaken your immune system, making it easier to get HIV and other infections.

A.5

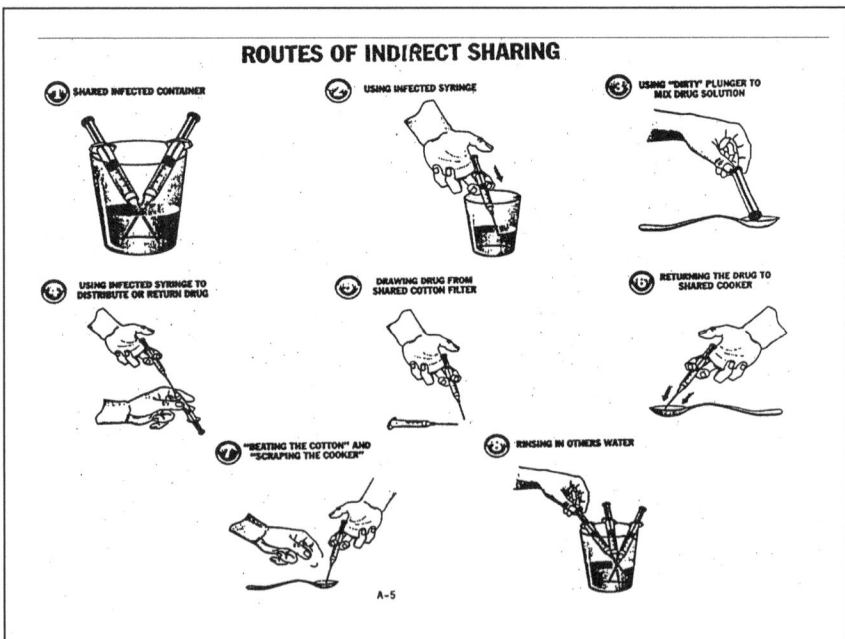

A.6

What about Cocaine and Crack?

- Sometimes people smoke crack or snort cocaine rather than inject it. But that doesn't mean they are safe. Even if they only smoke or snort, heavy cocaine users are still increasing their risk for HIV infection. Here's why:

  —People often have more sex when they use cocaine, and they often forget to wear latex condoms or to ask their partners to wear a condom.

  —Some people sell sex to get cocaine or to get money for cocaine. This may mean they have more sex or unprotected sex.

  —Crack and cocaine may weaken the immune system, making it easier to get HIV and other infections.

- If you are a crack or cocaine user, you can decrease your chances of getting HIV by getting off drugs.

- If you can't get off drugs, be sure to wear latex condoms or make sure your partners do. Your life depends on it!

A.7

Why Use Condoms?

- Condoms, used all the way through sex, help prevent the spread of sexually transmitted diseases including HIV, the virus that causes AIDS.

  —Lambskin, sheepskin, and other natural condoms do not protect you from HIV.

- Sexually transmitted diseases often cause lesions or sores. When these occur, it's easier to get infected with HIV.

- Besides not having sex, the best ways to protect yourself against AIDS are nonpenetrative sex or mutual masturbation (not oral sex). Using latex condoms is the next best way to protect yourself.

- For receiving oral sex, men should use condoms, and women should use dental dams or a barrier such as Saran Wrap.

- To reduce your risk of getting HIV/AIDS:
  Best method: no sex.
  Next best: no sex involving penetration.
  Next best: use condoms with all sex involving penetration.

- Spermicides like diaphragm jelly and contraceptive sponges do not kill HIV.

- Demonstration and rehearsal.

A.8

What about Female Condoms?

- Female condoms have been shown to reduce the risk of getting sexually transmitted diseases and pregnancy.

- Female condoms (like Reality) are polyurethane, baglike devices that are placed in the vagina to catch the male ejaculation (cum).

- Female and male condoms should never be used together at the same time.

- Each female condom can be used only one time. It must be thrown out after each sex act.

A.9

How to Talk with Your Partner about Safer Sex

- Learn as much as you can about HIV. That will make it easier to talk.

- Decide when you want to talk. The best time is not just before having sex.

- Decide in your own mind what you will and won't do during sex.

- Give your partner time to think about what you're saying. Don't rush.

- Pay attention to how your partner is understanding what you're saying. Slow down if you need to.

- Talk about the times that make it hard to have safe sex. These are times when you don't have condoms or have used alcohol or drugs. Try to decide what to do at those times so you can both be safe from HIV.

- If your partner does not want to practice safe sex, ask yourself if this is the type of person you really want to have sex with.

A.10

Why Clean Needles and Syringes?

- You can get infected with HIV by sharing works another person has used. You can also get HIV by sharing cookers, cotton, or rinse water.

- Merely rinsing used works in water, even hot water, will not kill HIV. You must use bleach.

- To reduce your risk of infection:
  Best method: stop using drugs.
  Next best: stop using needles.
  If you can't stop using needles, don't share needles. Use a new needle or a needle *only you* have used before.
  If you do share needles, clean the needle *every* time before you inject drugs. Clean it the way we are showing you today.

- Do not put your needle in someone else's rinse water, cotton, or cooker. HIV can live in blood in all these places.

- Demonstration and rehearsal.

A.11

Bleach, Bleach, Water, Water

- Always clean with full strength bleach.

- Keep bleach in syringe by tapping 30 seconds.

- Always discard into sink, toilet, or sewer.

- Bleach again.

- Always rinse with clean water and discard into sink, toilet, or sewer.

- Rinse again.

- After you finish with bleach, bleach, water, water, *then* remove plunger from syringe and clean both parts again with bleach and water.

- Never share your other equipment (cooker, cotton, cooking water, or rinse water).

- Clean your cooker with full strength bleach and rinse with clean water.

A.12

The Benefits of Drug Treatment

- Can help you get off drugs and teach you ways to stay off drugs.

- Can change your life, improve your health, and reduce your risk of HIV.

- Can provide counseling and support for you and family members who may also need help.

- Can provide referrals for other health and social services.

- Can provide support for dealing with AIDS and other problems.

- Even if you can't get into treatment now, you can be given informatoin on support groups that will help you until a treatment program can be found for you.

A.13

The HIV Test

- The test screens for the presence of antibodies that have developed in your system in response to the virus.

- A positive test shows that you are infected with HIV and can give it to others.

- A negative test may mean that you are free of the virus. There is a period of time between infection and when the test shows that you are infected. This is called the *window period*. During this time, you can test "negative" for HIV but you may really be "positive." It's a good idea to have another HIV test in 6 months to be sure you don't have the virus. (Between testing, if you have sex, make sure you use latex condoms. If you use needles, make sure you don't share works—use clean works.

- We recommend you take the text and learn your test results because
  —Treatment is available for HIV infection.
  —You can plan a course of action that is best for you, your family and friends, and your community.

- Some people are anxious about taking the HIV test or getting results. Our staff are prepared to discuss all concerns you may have about getting tested. Please feel free to ask any questions, so you can feel better about getting the test.

A.14

If You Are Infected with HIV

- It is important to get early medical treatment to control the disease.

- Be safe. Don't take in more virus—it can make you sicker. Do everything you can to reduce your risk.

- Some things you can do:
  —reduce drug use,
  —eat healthy foods,
  —get proper rest,
  —get proper exercise,
  —think positively, consider joining a support group,
  —get regular preventative medical care.

A.15

Partner Notification

- Partners may want to consider changing their behaviors, too.

- Partners may want to seek HIV testing and medical treatment if they are infected.

- The health department can help locate and counsel partners.

- Partner notification laws.

B.1

Meaning of Seronegative Results

- Negative results mean that HIV antibodies have not been found in the blood.

- Individuals who test negative may be infected with HIV. This can happen if your body hasn't yet produced enough antibodies to be detected.

- It usually takes 2 weeks to 6 months after you are infected for your body to produce a detectable level of antibodies. In a small number of people, it can take up to 3 years. A very small number of people never show antibodies, even though they are infected.

- Anyone who has engaged in risky behaviors in the last 6 months should be retested for HIV in the next 6 months. (Between testing, if you have sex, make sure you use latex condoms. If you use needles, make sure you don't share works—use clean works.)

- Anyone who has engaged in risky behaviors since 1977 should not donate or sell blood.

B.2

Meaning of Seropositive Results

- A person who tests positive is infected with the virus and can infect others.

- A person who tests positive may not have symptoms of AIDS. These symptoms may not develop for 5 to 10 years.

- People who are infected can take in more virus and get sicker unless they protect themselves with safe behaviors.

- The sexual partners, shooting buddies, or children of people who test positive may also be infected.

- A seropositive person should not donate or sell blood.

- A seropositive person should seek and receive regular medical care.

- A seropositive woman risks passing the virus to her fetus if she is pregnant and to her child if she is breast-feeding.

- Early medical treatment such as taking AZT may prevent passing the virus from mother to fetus.

C.1

Meaning of Seropositive Results

- A person who tests positive is infected with the virus and can infect others.

- A person who tests positive may not have symptoms of AIDS. These symptoms may not develop for 5 to 10 years.

- People who are infected can take in more virus and get sicker unless they protect themselves with safe behaviors.

- The sexual partners, shooting buddies, or children of people who test positive may also be infected.

- A seropositive person should not donate or sell blood.

- A seropositive person should seek and receive regular medical care.

- A seropositive woman risks passing the virus to her fetus if she is pregnant and to her child if she is breast-feeding.

- Early medical treatment such as taking AZT may prevent passing the virus from mother to fetus.

C.2

If You Are Infected with HIV

- Don't take in more of the virus by having unprotected oral, anal, or vaginal sex. Getting exposed to the virus again can make you sicker.

- Some things you can do: Stop using drugs. Reduce your number of sex partners. Get drug treatment. Join an HIV support group. Eat healthy foods. Get proper rest. Get proper exercise. Think positively. Get regular preventative medical care.

- Getting medical treatment is very important. Proper treatment can keep AIDS symptoms from developing as quickly as they would without it.

- Review local treatment resouces.

C.3

HIV Control Measures

To prevent spreading HIV to others, people with HIV should

- refrain from sexual intercourse unless condoms are used, and exercise caution when using condoms due to possible condom failure;

- not share needles or syringes, or any other drug-related equipment, paraphernalia, or works that may be contaminated with blood through previous use;

- not donate or sell blood, plasma, platelets, other blood products, semen, ova, tissues, organs, or breast milk—all of these things may contain HIV;

- have a skin test for tuberculosis; and

- notify future sexual partners of infection. (If the time of initial infection is known, notify persons with whom you have been sexual and needle partners since date of infection; and, if date of infection is unknown, notify persons with whom you have been sexual and needle partners for the previous year.

Appendix B
Unraveling the Concept of Race in Brazil

Brazilian and American scholars alike have spent much of the twentieth century studying the fluidity of race and its meaning in Brazil. Racial identities in Brazil are dynamic concepts that can be understood only if situated and explored within the appropriate cultural context. Empirical evidence of this fluidity of racial identification quickly came to the authors' attention within the context of the prevention initiative in Rio de Janeiro. Because the main objective of this program was to slow the spread of AIDS through client behavior change, comparisons of client data at the baseline and follow-up assessments formed the core analyses of the project. Through quality control procedures used to link client information collected at different points in time (such as matching on birth date, gender, and race), it was revealed that 62 clients, or 18.2 percent of the reassessment sample, had changed their racial self-identification. Our attempts to engage project staff in a dialogue about the fluidity of racial identity among these clients provided some insight into what might be called the "contextual redefinition" of race in Brazil. Within the context of this study, the ramifications of this phenomenon are clear. Racial comparisons of HIV risk, sexual activity, drug use, and behavioral change, which were part and parcel of U.S.-based research, would appear to be of little utility in this setting.

Theories of Race in Brazil

Anyone who says that Brazil is a racial paradise is not well-informed.
—*Carlos Hasenbalg, Rio de Janeiro, 1994*

The study of race and race-relations in Brazil is a complex undertaking and requires a thorough examination of both Brazilian culture and history. For American researchers to attempt an understanding of the complexities of race in Brazil, it is important to avoid the temptation of imposing an American system of racial classification on a starkly different cultural reality. Brazilian and American scholars alike have spent considerable time studying the concept of race and its evolution in Brazil. The result is a sizeable body of literature characterized by three basic schools of thought—"racial democracy," "racial revisionism," and "structuralism."

Racial Democracy

The notion that Brazil was a racial democracy was first posited by the noted Brazilian anthropologist Gilberto Freyre in the 1930s. Critical to the development of Freyre's racial democracy thesis was the idea that the original Portuguese colonizers had subscribed to a type of "racial exceptionalism," that is, looking beyond skin color and recognizing overall accomplishments (Hanchard 1994). Years of Moorish rule of the Iberian Peninsula, for example, had exposed the Portuguese to an advanced African civilization, and this was assumed to have created an acknowledgement of the worth and humanity of people of color. Furthermore, the widespread miscegenation that took place between the Portuguese colonizers and African slaves provided "proof" for early scholars of race relations that Brazil was in fact a racially egalitarian society.

By contrast, others have maintained that the slave system in Brazil was extremely cruel (Degler 1971). It has been estimated, for example, that 3.3 million slaves were supplied to Brazil, more than ten times the number received in the North American colonies (Wagley 1952). Other estimates placed the number as high as 4.5 million (Ellison 1995). By 1860, however, the slave population in Brazil was only about half that of North America, due to low fertility yet extremely high mortality rates. In fact, the Brazilian historian Decio Freitas estimated that the typical useful life span of a plantation slave was only five years. After abolition, however, high rates of intermarriage and the absence of racially discriminatory legislation, such as the Jim Crow laws of the American South, suggested to many that there was a favorable climate of race relations in Brazil and perpetuated the myth of a racial democracy. At least two important implications of the racial democracy thesis have been identified by social scientists: (1) the absence of racial prejudice and discrimination in Brazil (Hasenbalg 1985; Wood and Carvalho 1988); and (2) the relative unimportance of race in determining "life chances" (Wood and Carvalho 1988).

Racial Revisionism

As a response to the racial democracy model, scholars fostering a racial revisionism concept recognized the existence of prejudice in Brazil but viewed the issue as a class-based rather than race-based phenomenon (Hasenbalg 1985; Winant 1994). Acceptance by white society, in other words, was governed by class position and socioeconomic status rather than race or skin color (Wood and Carvalho 1988). It was also argued that the absence of a descent rule in Brazil through which race is inherited gives rise to dynamic racial identities and necessarily diminishes the importance of race relative to class (Harris et al. 1993). Although this perspective provided new insight into race relations in Brazil, it was limited by the refusal to recognize that race per se operates as a independent predictor of life chances (Winant 1994). The fact that income levels, employment, and educational achievement failed to equalize in the century after abolition, and that nonwhites remain concentrated in the bottom socioeconomic strata, all speak to the significance of race in Brazil.

The Structuralist Perspective

Recognition of the existence of racial prejudice and discrimination was a defining characteristic of the third line of research on Brazilian race relations. The structuralist perspective, and especially the work of Florestan Fernandes, a prominent sociologist associated with the "São Paulo school," examined the issue of race in terms of the transition from an agrarian slave society to an industrial one. Fernandes believed that racial prejudice and discrimination were requirements of a slave-based economy, but became dysfunctional in a capitalist, class-based economy. Furthermore, Carlos Hasenbalg, head of Afro-Asiatic studies at Cândido Mendes University in Rio de Janeiro, argued that racial discrimination obtained a new significance after abolition and became useful as a way to limit the opportunities of nonwhites for upward mobility (Hasenbalg 1985).

Whitening *and the "Mulatto Escape Hatch"*

Structuralists also sought to explain how the maintenance of racial inequalities had been accomplished so successfully without any large-scale resistance or opposition similar to the U.S. Civil Rights Movement of the 1960s. Within this context, Brazil is home to the largest black population in any nation outside of Africa, with an estimated 70 million residents of African descent. And, according to black activist leaders in Brazil, only about 25,000 are active participants in the National Black Movement (Burdick 1995). Proponents of the structuralist perspective have suggested that it was through the once official, but now defunct, Brazilian policy of "whitening" *(embranqueamento)* that racial inequalities have persisted virtually uncontested (Winant 1994). The "whitening" of the population through massive European immigration provided a large pool of relatively skilled white labor and prevented nonwhite Brazilians from obtaining a strong foothold in the labor market to gain bargaining power. Furthermore, in the face of the racist scientific doctrines of the late 1800s, which argued that blacks were both biologically and intellectually inferior, extensive racial miscegenation was encouraged in order to "whiten" the population and bring the racial composition of Brazil closer to the "ideal" (Wood and Carvalho 1988; Skidmore 1972).

North American sociologist Carl Degler (1971) offered an additional and somewhat complementary explanation for the minimally organized opposition to racial inequalities in Brazil in what he termed the "mulatto escape hatch." This proposition held that it was the greater social and economic opportunities granted to mulattoes that had prevented extensive racial divisions from taking root. According to this thesis, even blacks who may have had limited chances for mobility themselves were able to hope for much more for their children— through "miscegenation"—and therefore did not feel compelled to confront systemic racial inequality. Research data, however, have not supported the existence of a "mulatto escape hatch." Most studies suggest that blacks and mulattoes are equally represented among the lowest economic strata in Brazil (Winant 1994; Wood and Carvalho 1988). Qualitative research has documented, however, that among much of the Afro-Brazilian population the "mulatto escape hatch" phenomenon is perceived to be a reality, and may therefore have some relationship to the lack of racial polarization in Brazil.

Emic *and* Etic *Approaches to Racial Identity*

Because of the considerable racial ambivalence present in much of Brazilian society, a number of observers have suggested that an emic approach to the study of race in Brazil may be appropriate (Winant 1994; Harris et al. 1993). In contrast to the *etic* approach, which establishes racial identity through genetic testing and the rule of descent, the emic approach entails the use of people's categorizations of themselves and others to construct racial identities and meanings. Howard Winant (1994) embraced the emic approach to the study of race with the development of the "racial formation" perspective. This approach sees race not as a "natural" attribute, but one that is socially constructed and specific to a given society.

In the United States, racial groups are analogous to castes, in the sense that they are fixed identities inherited from parents and grandparents. As recently stated by the Brazilian scholar Marcelo Gentil:

> in the U.S., black is black and white is white. There is an open enmity which makes everything much easier (Ellison 1995).

In Brazil, however, it is the perception of phenotypical traits (skin color, hair texture, and facial features) that outweigh heritage to establish a racial identity (Harris et al. 1993; Haberly 1995).

The lack of a hard and fast rule for determining racial classification has led to the evolution of countless terms to denote color. In fact, one 1970 study reported that Brazilian respondents presented with 36 portraits of varied combinations of physical features used no less than 492 terms to describe race-color identity (Harris 1970). A similar survey a few years later garnered 143 color responses including gray, pink, *café au lait,* dirty white, corn, and cinnamon (Ellison 1995).

Context also plays an important role in race labeling (Harris et al. 1993; Haberly 1995), given the tendency in Brazil for racial identity to change according to class position. The well-known Brazilian expression, *"o dinheiro embranquece,"* or "money whitens," aptly communicates this idea that race and class are thoroughly intertwined. Racial terms may be used symbolically to signify wealth and social status (Hasenbalg and Huntington 1982). People with mixed physical characteristics may be labeled "white" if they appear well-dressed and occupy prestigious positions. Similarly, a poor mulatto may be labeled "black" to indicate social inferiority (Hasenbalg and Huntington 1982).

A remarkable example of this race/class phenomenon was described as part of a larger study of the Brazilian census (Harris et al. 1993). In the 1980 census, race had been categorized into a four-item choice: black, brown, white, or yellow. Interestingly, 54 percent of the respondents self-identified as *branca* (white), 38 percent as *parda* (brown), 6 percent as *preta* (black), and 2 percent as *amarela* (yellow). *"Parda"* was found to be an especially troublesome term because it had little meaning to the majority of Brazilians. The words most commonly used to designate "brown" among the general population were *morena* (brunette), *mulata* (mulatto), *morena clara* (light brunette), *cabo verde* (the color of those from the Cape Verde Islands), *clara* (fair), *sarará* (persons with kinky hair), and *escurinha* (a little dark). Only 37 percent of those who self-identified as *morena* in a free-choice interview later re-identified as *parda* in the four-item option. Respondents were equally as likely to re-identify as either white or black, according to the social position they occupied. From these data, the researchers concluded that census reports of the number of whites, browns, and blacks were distorted in the areas of Brazil they surveyed, and found it likely that similar confusion reigned for the nation as a whole. Others have echoed this sentiment, and regard the subjective nature of racial classification as an obstacle to reliable estimates of racial membership in Brazil (Haberly 1995).

Empirical Evidence of Racial Complexities

Empirical evidence of the fluidity and complexity of racial self-identification in Brazil quickly came to the authors' attention during the course of the HIV/AIDS prevention initiative described in this book. Fieldwork in Rio de Janeiro had begun in March 1994 and follow-up efforts were initiated in September of the same year. Through December 1995, reassessments had been completed on 341 clients. Because the main objective of the project was to slow the spread of AIDS through client behavior change, comparisons of client data at baseline and follow-up formed the core analyses of the project. Through quality control procedures used to link client information collected at the initial and subsequent assessments (such as matching on birth date, gender, and race), it was discovered that 62 clients, or 18.2 percent of the reassessment sample, had changed racial self-identification at follow-up:

- 11.3% from black to white;
- 37.1% from black to multiracial;
- 27.4% from white to multiracial;
- 6.4% from white to black;
- 8.1% multiracial to black; and,
- 9.7% multiracial to white.

Subsequent focus groups conducted with the project's interviewing staff offered several explanations for this phenomenon. The interviewers noted that as a rule, the clients (1) tended to place themselves in an "inferior" position during the interview, (2) seemed willing to agree and accept everything the interviewers asked of them, and (3) made an effort not to frustrate the interviewer. Consequently, they believe that clients may incorrectly identify their race as a "nondominant" one, especially on the first contact, in order to avoid offending the interviewer. The tendency of the clients to avoid placing themselves on the same level as the interviewer appears to be even stronger if the interviewer is white.

The interviewers also suggested that racial identification may shift at follow-up because the clients feel more at ease with the staff during subsequent contacts, and may be more honest in their responses. Alternative interpretations of the racial identity shift proposed in the focus groups included (1) an interaction between the level of intoxication (alcohol, cocaine) and racial identification, and (2) an interaction between the ethnicity and gender of the interviewer, his or her interviewing style, and racial identification.

Another issue revealed during the course of the interviewer focus groups that greatly impacted client racial identification was the imposition of U.S. racial categories on the interview schedule. Data collection instruments were standardized across the sites of the Cooperative Agreement and were developed for U.S. populations. The racial identification options included were "Black," "White," "Hispanic," "Asian," "Native American," and "Other." Of these, only "Black," "White," and "Other" are applicable to the vast majority of the residents of Rio de Janeiro. Many times, interviewer knowledge of the racial dichotomization that exists in the United States led to a situation of forced black or white self-identification, in an attempt to facilitate comparisons of Brazil and U.S. client data. Once the authors' became aware of this tendency in May 1995, the interviewers were instructed to allow the client to specify any racial identification that he or she wished. Although shifts in racial identification between baseline and follow-up have continued to occur at nearly the same rate since this change was made, the proportion of the sample identifying as multiracial has jumped dramatically. Through May 1995 only 9.8 percent of the clients had self-identified as multiracial, however by December 1995, this proportion had increased to 26.5 percent. More specifically, and as indicated in Figure B.1, especially significant changes occurred immediately after clients were instructed to self-identify as they wished.

An analysis of the shifts in self-identification yielded the following:

1. Male clients were overwhelmingly more likely than female clients to change their racial identification ($p=.004$). Of the 62 race changers, only 1 was a woman. There was no relationship between client and interviewer gender and/or race.
2. At baseline, clients were significantly more likely ($p=.02$) to identify as multiracial if interviewed by a male.
3. At follow-up, the significant trend ($p=.000$) was to identify as multiracial, in that 64.5% of race changers changed to multiracial. Interestingly, there was no *significant* relationship between baseline identification and changing race. But, at baseline, 48.4% of race changers identified as black, 33.9% as white, 17.7% as multiracial.
4. Clients interviewed by white interviewers at the first contact were more likely to change race at follow-up than clients interviewed by black interviewers ($p=.05$), in that 20.6% of clients interviewed by whites changed compared to 11.7% of clients interviewed by blacks.
5. Clients interviewed by males (at follow-up) were more likely to change racial identification than clients interviewed by females ($p=.02$)

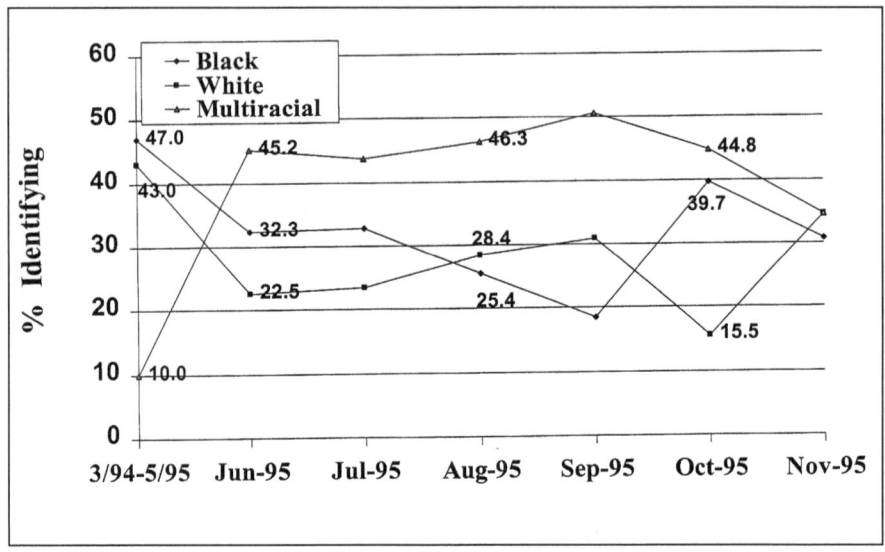

FIGURE B.1   Respondent Racial Self-Identification by Month,Rio de Janeiro

Discussion

Brazil has always cherished its image as a paradise of racial equality. Segregation laws have never existed in Brazil, and any kind of discrimination is illegal. Yet the ideology that everyone is the same is a myth. Most black Brazilians recognize that they are victims of discrimination, but the racism appears to be quite subtle. Or as Robert Ananias of the Rio Council on Race Relations recently stated: "Here they hug you while they stab you in the back" (Goering 1994). At the same time, racial identity is fragmented, a phenomenon that is well documented in the intervention study data.

Although the data gathered during the research process by no means represent a comprehensive study of race in Brazil, they do support much of what is known about the nature of social interactions in Brazil. The notions of class and position are very strong in Brazil and tend to influence a variety of life choices. Jobs are typically accorded a particular status, and members of the upper or middle classes would not normally take on a lower class function. For example, upper and upper-middle-class women who choose to work after or instead of college would probably not accept a secretarial position because it lacks a certain status (Harrison 1995).

As one might expect in such a system of social organization, cross-class interactions are few, with the exception of specific role performances such as employer and maid. Often, even language reflects this hierarchical class system. Dr. Phyllis Harrison (1995), author of *Behaving Brazilian*, noted that it is commonplace to hear the phrase *"Você sabe com quem está falando?"* ("Do you know who you're talking to?") uttered by an upper-class Brazilian when sensing disrespect from a member of the lower class. Similarly, a person of lower status may address a person of higher rank as *"doutor"* (doctor), regardless of educational degrees, in order to show social deference. Within this context, our attempts to engage project staff in a dialogue about the fluidity of racial identity among our clients may indeed have shed some light on what might be called the "contextual redefinition" of race. The virtually universal membership of our client population in the lowest echelons of Brazilian society and their persistent references to project staff as *"doutor"* demonstrated that a perception of social distance was present during the interview session. This may offer some support for the interviewers' assertions that the clients chose to identify their race as a "nondominant" one, particularly in interactions with white interviewers.

Certainly, the reasons for the observed shifts in racial identity remain unclear, and only further monitoring and analysis will provide additional insight into the interaction of race, class, and gender that appears to be at work. What is apparent to those of us engaged in research on drug use and HIV, however, is the limited utility of "race" in Brazil as a construct for analysis. At many U.S.-based project sites, race was one of the most significant and consistent predictors of HIV risk and serostatus. In contrast, any attempt to discern racial differences in Rio study data—including HIV risk, sexual activity, drug use, and behavioral changes—appeared to be of little utility.

References

Chapter 1

Baden, M.M. (1975) "Methadone Related Deaths in New York City," *International Journal of the Addictions*, 5:489–498.

Bond, G.C., J. Kreniske, I. Susser, and J. Vincent (1997) *AIDS in Africa and the Caribbean* (Boulder: Westview Press).

Browning, F. (1993) *The Culture of Desire: Paradox and Perversity in Gay Lives Today* (New York: Crown Publishers).

Centers for Disease Control (1981a) "Pneumocystis Pneumonia—Los Angeles," *Morbidity and Mortality Weekly Report*, 30 (5 June):250–252.

Centers for Disease Control (1981b) "Kaposi's Sarcoma and Pneumocystis Pneumonia among Homosexual Men—New York City and California," *Morbidity and Mortality Weekly Report*, 30 (3 July):305–308.

Centers for Disease Control (1982) "Epidemiologic Aspects of the Current Outbreak of Kaposi's Sarcoma and Opportunistic Infections," *New England Journal of Medicine*, 306:248–252.

Edwards, S. and C. Carne (1998) "Oral Sex and the Transmission of Viral STIs," *Sexually Transmitted Infections*, 74:6–10.

Fischl, M.A., G.M. Dickenson, G.B. Scott, N. Klimas, M. A. Fletcher, and W. Parks (1987) "Evaluation of Heterosexual Partners, Children, and Household Contacts of Adults with AIDS," *Journal of the American Medical Association*, 257:640–644.

Giudici-Fettner, A. (1987) "The Discovery of AIDS: Perspectives from a Medical Journalist," in G.P. Wormser, R.E. Stahl, and E.J. Bottone (eds.), *AIDS and Other Manifestations of HIV Infection* (Park Ridge, NJ: Noyes Publications), pp. 2–17.

Goedert, J.J., M.E. Eyster, M.V. Ragni, R.J. Biggar, and M.H. Gail (1988) "Rate of Heterosexual Transmission and Associated Risk with HIV Antigen," *IV International Conference on AIDS*, Stockholm, Sweden, June 12–18.

Golden, J.A. (1989) "Pulmonary Complications of AIDS," in J.A. Levy (ed.), *AIDS: Pathogenesis and Treatment* (New York: Marcel Dekker), pp. 403–447.

Gordis, E. (1992) "Alcohol and AIDS," National Institute on Alcohol Abuse and Alcoholism, *Alcohol Alert*, 15 (January).

Gottlieb, M.S., R. Schroff, H. Schanker, J.D. Weismal, P.T. Fan, R.A. Wolf, and A. Saxon (1981) "Pneumocystis Carinii Pneumonia and Mucosal Candidiasis in Previously Healthy Homosexual Men: Evidence of a New Acquired Cellular Immunodeficiency," *New England Journal of Medicine*, 305:1425–1431.

Grund, J.P.C., C.D. Kaplan, N.F.P. Adriaans, P. Blanken, and J. Huisman (1990) "The Limitations of the Concept of Needle Sharing: The Practice of Frontloading," *AIDS*, 4:819–821.

Holmberg, S.D., C.R. Horsburg, J.W. Ward, and H.W. Jaffe (1989) "Biological Factors in the Heterosexual Transmission of Human Immunodeficiency Virus," *Journal of Infectious Diseases*, 160:116–125.

Hughes, W.T. (1979) "Pneumocystis Carinii," in G.L. Mandell, R. G. Douglous, and J. E. Bennett (eds.), *Principles and Practices of Infectious Diseases* (New York: John Wiley), pp. 2137–2142.

Inciardi, J.A. (1990) "AIDS—A Strange Disease of Uncertain Origins," *American Behavioral Scientist*, 33:397–407.

Inciardi, J.A. (1992) *The War on Drugs II: The Continuing Epic of Heroin, Cocaine, Crack, Crime, AIDS, and Public Policy* (Mountain View, CA: Mayfield).

Inciardi, J.A. and J.B. Page (1991) "Drug Sharing among Intravenous Drug Users," *AIDS*, 5:772–774.

Institute of Medicine (1986) *Mobilizing Against AIDS: The Unfinished Story of a Virus* (Cambridge: Harvard University Press).

Johnson, A.M. and M. Laga (1988) "Heterosexual Transmission of HIV," *AIDS*, 2 (suppl. 1):S49-S56.

Johnson, A., A. Petherick, S. Davison, S. Howard, L. Osborne, C. Sonnex, R. Robertson, S. Tchamouroff, M. Hooker, R. Brettle, and M.W. Adler (1988) "Transmission of HIV to Heterosexual Partners of Infected Men and Women," *IV International Conference on AIDS*, Stockholm, Sweden, June 12–18.

Kaplan, J. (1983) *The Hardest Drug: Heroin and Public Policy* (Chicago: University of Chicago Press).

Laga, M., H. Taelman, L. Bonneux, P. Cornet, G. Vercauteren, and P. Piot (1988) "Risk Factors for Heterosexual Partners of HIV-Infected Africans and Europeans," *IV International Conference on AIDS*, Stockholm, Sweden, June 12–18.

Louria, D.B. (1970) "Sexual Use of Amyl Nitrite," *Medical Aspects of Human Sexuality*, 4:89.

Martin, L.S., J.S. McDougal, and S.L. Lsokoski (1985) "Disinfection and Inactivation of the Human T Lymphotropic Virus Type III/ Lymphadenopathy-Associated Virus," *Journal of Infectious Diseases*, 152:400–403.

Masur, H., M.A. Michelis, J.B. Greene, I. Onorato, R.A., Vande Stouwe, R.T. Holzman, G. Wormser, L. Brettmen, M. Lange, H.W. Murray, and S. Cunningham-Rundles (1981) "An Outbreak of Community-Acquired Pneumocystis Carinii Pneumonia: Initial Manifestation of Cellular Immune Dysfunction," *New England Journal of Medicine*, 305:1431–1438.

McCoy, C.B. and J.A. Inciardi (1995) *Sex, Drugs, and the Continuing Spread of AIDS* (Los Angeles: Roxbury).

Nickerson, M. (1975) "Vasodilator Drugs," in L.S. Goodman and A. Gilman (eds.), *The Pharmacological Basis of Therapeutics* (New York: Macmillan), pp. 727–743.

Padian, N., J. Wiley, S. Glass, L. Marquis, and W. Winkelstein (1988) "Anomalies of Infectivity in the Heterosexual Transmission of HIV," *IV International Conference on AIDS*, Stockholm, Sweden, June 12–18.

Parker, R. G. (1991) *Bodies, Pleasures and Passions: Sexual Culture in Contemporary Brazil* (Boston: Beacon Press).

Peterman, T.A., R.L. Stoneburner, J.R. Allen, H.W. Jaffe, and J.W. Curran (1988) "Risk of Human Immunodeficiency Transmission from Heterosexual Adults with Transfusion Associated Infections," *Journal of the American Medical Association*, 259:55–58.

Polk, B.F., R. Fox, R. Brookmeyer, S. Kanchanaraksa, R. Kaslow, B. Visscher, C. Rinalso, and J. Phair (1987) "Predictors of Acquired Immunodeficiency Syndrome Developing in a Cohort of Seropositive Homosexual Men," *New England Journal of Medicine*, 316:61–66.

Resnick, L.K, S.Z. Veren, S. Salahuddin, S. Tondreau, and P.D. Karkham (1986) "Stability and Inactivation of HTLV-III/LAV under Clinical and Laboratory Environments," *Journal of the American Medical Association*, 255:1887–1891.

Rompalo, A. and H.H. Handsfield (1989) "Overview of Sexually Transmitted Diseases in Homosexual Men," in P. Ma and D. Armstrong, (eds.), *AIDS and Infections of Homosexual Men* (Boston: Butterworths), pp. 3–11.

Seymour, R. and D.E. Smith (1987) *Guide to Psychoactive Drugs* (New York: Harrington Park Press).

Shapshak, P., C.B. McCoy, S.M. Shah, J.B. Page, J.E. Rivers, N.L. Weatherby, D.D. Chitwood, and D.C. Mash (1994) "Preliminary Laboratory Studies of Inactivation of HIV–1 in Needles and Syringes Containing Infected Blood Using Undiluted Household Bleach," *Journal of Acquired Immune Deficiency Syndromes*, 7:754–759.

Silverstein, C. and F. Picano (1992) *The New Joy of Gay Sex* (New York: Harper Collins).

United Nations Program on HIV/AIDS (1998) *AIDS Epidemic Update* (Geneva: UNAIDS).

Vogt, M.W., D.J. Witt, D. Craven, R. Byington, D. Crawford, M.S. Hutchinson, R.T. Schooley, and M.S. Hirsch (1987) "Isolation Patterns of the Human Immunodeficiency Virus from Cervical Secretions During the Menstrual Cycle of Women at Risk for the Acquired Immunodeficiency Syndrome," *Annals of Internal Medicine*, 106:380–382.

Winkelstein, W., N.S. Padian, G. Rutherford, and H.F. Jaffe (1989) "Homosexual Men," in R.A. Kaslow and D.P. Francis (eds.), *The Epidemiology of AIDS: Expression, Occurrence, and Control of Human Immunodeficiency Virus Type 1 Infection* (New York: Oxford University Press), pp. 117–135.

World Health Organization (1999) "Global AIDS Surveillance," *Weekly Epidemiological Record*, 47 (26 November):401–402.

Chapter 2

Bethell, L. (1987) *Colonial Brazil* (Cambridge: Cambridge University Press).

Burns, E.B. (1980) *A History of Brazil* (New York: Columbia University Press).

Conselho de Entorpecentes do Distrito Federal (1995) *Levantamento Sobre Consumo e Causas que Levam os Estudantes ao Uso de Drogas* (Brasília: GDF—SE-Fundação Educacional).

Dunn, J. and R. Laranjeira (1999) "Cocaine B Profiles, Drug Histories, and Patterns of Use of Patients from Brazil," *Substance Use and Misuse*, 34(11): 1527–1548.

Eisenstien, E. (1992) *Street Youth. Rio de Janeiro: Nucleo de Estudos e Pesquisas Em Atenção de Drogas*. Unpublished paper.

Foucault, M. (1978) *The History of Sexuality: An Introduction* (New York: Random House).

Freyre, G. (1986) *The Mansions and the Shanties; the Making of Modern Brazil* (Berkeley: University of California Press).

Fagundes, R. (1997) "Rota Marcada de Dor," *Jornal do Brasil*, August 24, p. 8.

Guerra de Andrade, A. (1995) "As Drogas Mais Usadas no Brasil e Suas Conseqüências," in Ministério da Saúde (ed.) *Drogas, AIDS e Sociedade* (Brasília: Ministério da Saúde), pp. 55–59.

International Child Resource Institute (1994) *Brazil Street Children Bulletin*, Summer:1–3.

Latinamerica Press (1996) "The Three Faces of Brazil," 28 (July 25):4–5.

Martins, J.P.S. (1993) "Children in Brazil victims through the ages," *Latinamerica Press* (December 23):4.

Michaels, M. (1993) "Rio's Dead End Kids," *Time*, 142(August 9):36–37.

Parker, R. (1986) "Masculinity, Femininity, and Homosexuality: On the Anthropological Interpretation of Sexual Meanings in Brazil," *Journal of Homosexuality*, 11:155–163.

Parker, R. (1991) *Bodies, Pleasures, Passions: Sexual Cultures in Contemporary Brazil* (Boston: Beacon Press).

Parker, R. (1999) *Beneath the Equator: Cultures of Desire, Male Homosexuality, and Emerging Gay Communities in Brazil* (New York: Routledge).

Raphael, A. and J. Berkman (1992) "Children Without a Future," *Brazil Network* (September):1–35.

Surratt, H.L. and P.R. Telles (1999) "The Harm Reduction Movement in Brazil," in J.A. Inciardi and L.D. Harrison (eds.), *Harm Reduction: National and International Perspectives* (Newbury Park, CA: Sage Publications), pp.137–153.

Tilak, J. (1989) "Education and Its Relation to Economic Growth, Poverty, and Income Distribution: Past Evidence and Further Analysis," in *World Bank Discussion Paper No. 46* (Washington, DC: World Bank).

Uchôa, M.A. (1996) *Crack: O Caminho das Pedras* (São Paulo: Editora Ática).

United Nations Children's Fund (UNICEF) (1996) *Country Profile: Brazil* (Geneva: UNICEF).

Willumsen, M.J.F. and E. Giannetti da Fonseca (1997) *The Brazilian Economy: Structure and Performance in Recent Decades* (Miami: University of Miami North-South Center Press).

Wood, C.H. and J.A. Magno de Carvalho (1988) *The Demography of Inequality in Brazil* (New York: Cambridge University Press).

Chapter 3

Bastos, F.I., C. Lopes, P.R. Dias, E.S. Lima, and S.B. Luz (1988) "Perfil de Usuários de Drogas I," *Revista ABP-APAL*, 10: 47–52.

Brazilian Ministry of Health (1995) *Boletim Epidemiológico AIDS*, 8(2):March/May.

Brazilian Ministry of Health (1999) *Boletim Epidemiologic AIDS*, 12(2):March/May.

Cortes, E., R. Deters, D. Aboulafia, S. Li, D. Slamon, and D. Ho (1989a) "Seroprevalence of HIV–1, HIV–2, and HTLV–1 in Male Prostitutes in Rio de Janeiro, Brazil," *V International Conference on AIDS*, Montreal, June 4–9.

Cortes E., R. Deters, D. Slamon, D. Aboulafia, X.L. Li, and D.D. Ho (1989b) "Study of HIV–1, HIV–2 and HTLV–1 in Female Prostitutes in Brazil," *V International Conference on AIDS*, Montreal, June 4–9.

Daniel, H. and R. Parker (1993) *Sexuality, Politics, and AIDS in Brazil* (London: Falmer Press).

Guillermoprieto, A. (1990) *Samba* (New York: Alfred A. Knopf).

Guimarães, M., E. Castilho, and C.R. Filho (1991) "Heterosexual Transmission of HIV: A Multicenter Study in Rio de Janeiro," *VII International Conference on AIDS*, Florence, June 16–21.

Inciardi, J.A. (1986) The War on Drugs: Heroin, Cocaine, Crime, and Public Policy (Palo Alto, CA: Mayfield Publishing).

Inciardi, J.A. and R.H. Needle (1998) "HIV/AIDS Interventions for Out-of-Treatment Drug Users," *Journal of Psychoactive Drugs*, 30(3):225–229.

Lima, E.S., P.R. Dias, F.I. Bastos, and C. Lopes (1990) "Perfil de Usuários de Drogas: Danos a Integridade Física e Psicosocial," *Informação Psiquiatrica*, 9:117–120.

Lima, E.S., F.I. Bastos, and S.R. Friedman (1991) "HIV–1 Epidemiology among IVDUs in Rio de Janeiro, Brazil," *VII International Conference on AIDS*, Florence, June 16–21.

Lima, E.S., F.I. Bastos, P.R. Telles, and S.R. Friedman (1993) "HIV Infection and AIDS among Drug Injectors at Rio de Janeiro: Perspectives and Unanswered Questions," *Bulletin on Narcotics*, 45(1):107–115.

Masur, J. and B.C. Cotrim (1987) "Padrão de Uso de Drogas Psicotropicas Precedendo a Internação por Dependência," *Revista Brasileira de Psiquiatria*, 9:145–150.

Monteiro, M.G. and J.A. Inciardi (1993) *Brasil–United States Binational Research* (São Paulo, Brasil: CEBRID).

Parker, R. (1999) *Beneath the Equator* (New York: Routledge).

Quinn, T.C., J.P. Narain, and R.K. Zacarais (1990) "AIDS in the Americas: A Public Health Priority for the Region," *AIDS*, 4:709–724.

Rodrigues, L. and P. Chequer (1989) "AIDS in Brazil," *PAHO Bulletin*, 23:30–34.

Telles, P., F. Bastos, E. Lima, S. Friedman, and D. Des Jarlais (1992) "HIV–1 Epidemiology among IDUs in Rio de Janeiro, Brazil," *VIII International Conference on AIDS*, Amsterdam, July 19–24.

Telles, P., F. Bastos, F. Mesquita, R. Stall, N. Hearst, and R. Bueno (1994) "Assessing Risk Behaviors and HIV Seroprevalence among IDUs in Two Major Ports of South America," *X International Conference on AIDS*, Yokohama, August 7–12.

Watters, J.K. and P. Biernacki (1989) "Targeted Sampling: Options for the Study of Hidden Populations," *Social Problems*, 36:416–430.

World Health Organization (1999) *Weekly Epidemiological Record*, 74(47):401–408.

Chapter 4

AIDSCAP (1996) *Behavior Change: A Summary of Four Major Theories*, AIDSCAP Behavioral Research Unit.

Ankrah, E.M. (1991) "AIDS and the Social Side of Health," *Social Science and Medicine*, 32(9):967–980.

Barbosa de Carvalho, H., F. Mesquita, E. Massad, R.C. Bueno, G.T. Lopes, M.A. Ruiz, and M. Burattini (1996) "HIV and Infections of Similar Transmission Patterns in a Drug Injectors Community of Santos, Brazil," *Journal of Acquired Immune Deficiency Syndromes and Human Retrovirology*, 12:84–92.

Brazilian Ministry of Health (1998) *Global and Regional Summaries of the HIV/ AIDS/STD Epidemics* <www.aids.gov.br/udtv/map_global.htm>.

Daniel, H. and R. Parker (1993) *Sexuality, Politics, and AIDS in Brazil* (Bristol, PA: The Falmer Press).

Guillermoprieto, A. (1990) *Samba* (New York: Alfred A. Knopf).

Inciardi, J.A. (1986) *The War on Drugs: Heroin, Cocaine, Crime, and Public Policy* (Palo Alto, CA: Mayfield Publishing).

Inciardi, J.A. and H.L. Surratt (2000) "An AIDS Risk Reduction Model for Young Adult Cocaine Users in Brasil," Health Promotion in the Americas: Theory and practice. Pan American Health Organization (in press).

Inciardi, J.A., H.L. Surratt, and H.V. McCoy (1997) "Establishing an HIV/AIDS Intervention Program for Street Drug Users in a Developing Nation," *Journal of Drug Issues*, 27(1):173–193.

Krueger, L.E., R.W. Wood, P.H. Dehr, and G.L. Maxwell (1990) "Poverty and HIV Seropositivity: The Poor Are More Likely to Be Infected with AIDS," *AIDS*, 4:811–814.

Males, M. (1996) "AIDS and Ethnicity," *Science*, 271:1479–1480.

Montoya, I.D., A. Richard, D. Bell, and J. Atkinson (1997) "An Analysis of Unmet Need for HIV Services: The Houston Study," *Journal of Health Care for the Poor and Underserved*, 8(4):446–460.

McBride, D.C., N.L. Weatherby, J.A. Inciardi, and S. Gillespie (1999) "AIDS Susceptibility in a Migrant Population: Perception and Behavior," *Substance Use and Misuse*, 34(4 and 5):633–652.

Rambali, P. (1993) *In the Cities and Jungles of Brazil* (New York: Henry Holt and Company).

Rosenstock, I., V. Strecher, and M. Becker (1994) "The Health Belief Model and HIV Risk Behavior Change," in R.J. DiClemente and J.L. Peterson (eds.), *Preventing AIDS: Theories and Methods of Behavioral Interventions* (New York: Plenum Press).

Scholl, P. (1997) *The Favela's Relationship to the Environment and Urban Concepts.* Unpublished report.

Telles, P.R., F.I. Bastos, J. Guydish, J.A. Inciardi, H.L. Surratt, M. Pearl, and N. Hearst (1997) "Risk Behavior and HIV Seroprevalence among Injecting Drug Users in Rio de Janeiro, Brazil," *AIDS*, 11(suppl 1):S35-S42.

United Nations Programme on HIV/AIDS (1998) *Report on the Global HIV/AIDS Epidemic*, June.

Walton, R. (1990) "HIV infection and AIDS: Another Layer to Consider in Addressing Indigent Health Care in the United States," *Journal of Health and Social Policy*, 2(1):35–45.

Wechsberg, W.M., B.R. MacDonald, M.L. Dennis, J.A. Inciardi, H.L. Surratt, C.G. Leukefeld, D. Farrabee, L.B. Cottler, W.M. Compton, J.Hoffman, H. Klein, D. Desmond, and B. Zule (1997) *The Standard Intervention for Reduction in HIV Risk Behavior: Protocol Changes Suggested by the Continuing HIV/AIDS Epidemic* (Bloomington, IL: Chestnut Health Systems).

Zierler S. and N. Krieger (1997) "Reframing Women's Risk: Social Inequalities and HIV Infection," *Annual Review Public Health*, 18:401–436.

Chapter 5

Affonso, R. (1997) "A Final, Que Coador é Esse," *Jornal do Brasil*, Mulher, August 9, pp.1–2.

Ashery, R.S., R.G. Carlson, R.S. Falck, H.A. Siegal, and J. Wang (1995) "Female Condom Use among Injection Drug and Crack Cocaine-Using Women," *American Journal of Public Health*, 85:736–737.

Berkley, S. (1993) "AIDS in the Developing World: An Epidemiologic Overview," *Clinical Infectious Diseases*, 17(suppl. 2):S329-S336.

Blumenfeld, L. (1992) "The New Sexual 'Reality'," *The Washington Post*, March 9.

Bounds, W. (1989) "Male and Female Condoms," *British Journal of Family Planning*, 15:14–17.

Bounds, W., J. Guillebaud, L. Stewart, and S. Steele (1988) "A Female Condom (Femshield): A Study of Its User Acceptability," *The British Journal of Family Planning*, 14:83–87.

Brazilian Ministry of Health (1999) *Boletim Epidemiologico AIDS*, 12(2): March/May.

Calsyn, D.A., A.J. Saxon, E.A. Wells, and D.M. Greenberg (1992) "Longitudinal Sexual Behavior Changes in Injecting Drug Users," *AIDS* 6: 1207–1211.

Campbell, C. (1990) "Women and AIDS," *Social Science and Medicine*, 30:407–415.

Carovano, K. (1991) "More Than Mothers and Whores: Redefining the AIDS Prevention Needs of Women," *International Journal of Health Services*, 21:131–142.

Center for Reproductive Law and Policy (1995) *Brazil: STDs and HIV/AIDS*. Discussion paper.

Drew, W.L., M. Blair, R.C. Miner, and M. Conant (1989) *Evaluation of the Virus Permeability of a New Condom for Women*. Unpublished manuscript from the Mount Zion Hospital and Medical Center, Biskind Pathology Research Laboratory and the University of California, San Francisco.

Editorial (1992) "The female condom," *British Journal of Family Planning*, 18:71–72.

Gay, R. (1994) *Popular Organization and Democracy in Rio de Janeiro: A Tale of Two Favelas* (Philadelphia, PA: Temple University Press).

Goldberg, H.I., N.C. Lee, M.W. Oberle, and H.B. Peterson (1989) "Knowledge about Condoms and Their Use in Less Developed Countries During a Period of Rising AIDS Prevalence," *Bulletin of the World Health Organization*, 67:85–91.

Goldstein, D. (1994) "AIDS and Women in Brazil: The Emerging Problem," *Social Science and Medicine*, 39:919–929.

Gollub, E.L. and Z.A. Stein (1993) "Commentary: The New Female Condom— Item I on a Women's AIDS Prevention Agenda," *American Journal of Public Health*, 83:498–500.

Guillermoprieto, A. (1990) *Samba* (New York: Alfred A. Knopf).

Gupta, G.R. and E. Weiss (1993) "Women's Lives and Sex: Implications for AIDS Prevention," *Culture, Medicine, and Psychiatry*, 17:399–412.

Heise, L. and C. Elias (1995) "Transforming AIDS Prevention to Meet Women's Needs: A Focus on Developing Countries," *Social Science and Medicine*, 40:931–943.

Hernandez-Avila, M. (1992) *Acceptability of the Female Condoms among Female Prostitutes in Mexico City: Preliminary Findings*. Unpublished letter to Dr. Mary Ann Leeper from Dr. Mauricio Hernandez-Avila, director, Center for Public Health Research, National Institute of Public Health, Mexico.

Hetherington, S.E., R.M. Harris, R.B. Bausell, K.H. Kavanagh, and D.E. Scott (1996) "AIDS Prevention in High-Risk African-American Women: Behavioral, Psychological, and Gender Issues," *Journal of Marital and Sex Therapy*, 22(1):9–21.

Inciardi, J.A. and H.L. Surratt (1995) "Use of the Female Condom for Anal Sex," *III National Conference of Transvestites and the Liberated*, Rio de Janeiro, Brazil, June 13–16.

Inciardi, J.A., H.L. Surratt, and R. Ferreira de Melo (1997) "O Preservativo Feminino," *Revista Brasileira de Medicina Ginecologia e Obstetrícia*, 8(1):38–40.

Jackson, L. (1994) "The Female Condom Gets Mixed Reviews," *Philadelphia Daily News*, October 18, pp.4.

Leeper, M.A. (1990) "Preliminary Evaluation of Reality: A Condom for Women to Wear," *AIDS Care*, 2(3):287–290.

Leeper, M.A. and M. Conrardy (1989) "Preliminary Evaluation of Reality: A Condom for Women to Wear," *Advances in Contraception*, 5:229–235.

Loveman, B. (1991) "Latin America Faces Public Enemy No.1," *Institute of the American Hemisfile*, 2(July):6–8.

McBride, D.C., N.L. Weatherby, J.A. Inciardi, and S.A. Gillespie (1997) "AIDS Susceptibility in a Migrant Population: Perception and Behavior," *125th Annual Meeting of the American Public Health Association*, Indianapolis, Indiana, November 17–20.

Potts, M. and R.V. Short (1989) "Condoms for the Prevention of HIV Transmission: Cultural Dimensions," *AIDS*, 3(suppl 1): S259–S263.

Sacco, W.P., B. Levine, D.L. Reed, and K. Thompson (1991) "Attitudes about Condom Use as an AIDS-Relevant Behavior: Their Factor Structure and Relation to Condom Use," *Psychological Assessment: A Journal of Consulting and Clinical Psychology*, 3:265–272.

Sakondhavat, C. (1990) "Further Testing of Female Condoms," *British Journal of Family Planning*, 15:129.

Schilling, R.F., N. El-Bassel, M.A. Leeper, and L. Freeman (1991) "Acceptance of the Female Condom by Latin- and African-American Women," *American Journal of Public Health*, 81:1345–1346.

Scholl, P. (1997) "Family Organization in the Favela: Sexuality, Maternal and Paternal Feelings," Unpublished report. HIV/AIDS Community Outreach in Rio de Janeiro, Brazil.

Shervington, D.O. (1993) "The Acceptability of the Female Condom among Low-Income African-American Women," *Journal of the National Medical Association,* 85:341–347.

Sly, D.F., D. Quadagno, D.F. Harrison, I.W. Eberstein, K. Riehman, and M. Bailey (1997) Factors Associated with Use of the Female Condom," *Family Planning Perspectives,* 29(4):181–184.

Soper, D.E., N.J. Brockwell, and H.P. Dalton (1991) "Evaluation of the Effects of a Female Condom on the Female Lower Genital Tract," *Contraception,* 44(1): 21–29.

Soper, D.E., D. Shoupe, G.A. Shangold, M.M. Shangold, J. Gutmann, and L. Mercer (1993) "Prevention of Vaginal Trichomoniasis by Compliant Use of the Female Condom," *Sexually Transmitted Diseases,* (in press).

Stein, Z. (1990) "HIV prevention: The Need for Methods Women Can Use," *American Journal of Public Health,* 80:460–462.

Stein, Z.A. (1995) "Editorial: More on Women and the Prevention of HIV Infection," *American Journal of Public Health,* 85:1485–1488.

Surratt, H.L. and J.A. Inciardi (1999) "Introducing the Female Condom to Drug users in Brazil," *Population Research and Policy Review,* 18:169–181.

Surratt, H.L., P.R. Telles, and J.A. Inciardi (1999) "O uso do Preservativo Feminino entre Usuárias de Drogas no Rio de Janeiro," *Revista da ABEAD,* June(1): 9–19.

Surratt, H.L., W. Wechsberg, L. Cottler, C. Leukefeld, H. Klein, and D. Desmond (1998) "Acceptability of the Female Condom among Women at Risk for HIV Infection," *American Behavioral Scientist,* 41(8):1157–1170.

Valdiserri, R.O., V.C. Arena, D. Proctor, and F.A. Bonati (1989) "The Relationship between Women's Attitudes about Condoms and Their Use: Implications for Condom Promotion Programs," *American Journal of Public Health,* 79:499–501.

Voeller, B. (1991) "Gas, Dye, and Viral Transport Through Polyurethane Condoms," *Journal of the American Medical Association,* 266(21):2986–2987.

World Health Organization (1997) "Global AIDS Surveillance," *Weekly Epidemiologic Record,* 72:197–204.

World Health Organization Global Programme on AIDS (1995) *Women and AIDS: Agenda for Action,* September 28.

Worth, D. (1989) "Sexual Decision-Making and AIDS: Why Condom Promotion among Vulnerable Women Is Likely to Fail," *Studies in Family Planning,* 20:297–307.

Chapter 6

Bloom, P.(1997) *Brazil Up Close* (Edison, NJ: Hunter).

Box, B.(1994) *South American Handbook* (Chicago: NTC Publishing Group).

Box, B.(1997) *South American Handbook* (Chicago: NTC Publishing Group).

Bullough, V.L. and B. Bullough (1993) *Cross Dressing, Sex, and Gender* (Philadelphia: University of Pennsylvania Press).

Daniel,H. and R.G. Parker (1993) *Sexuality, Politics, and AIDS in Brazil* (London: Falmer Press).

Docter, R.F. (1988) *Transvestites and Transsexuals: Toward a Theory of Cross-Gender Behavior* (New York: Plenum Press).

Docter, R.F. and V. Prince (1997) "Transvestism: A Survey of 1032 Cross-Dressers," *Archives of Sexual Behavior*, 26: 589–605.

Ellis, H. (1926) *Eonism and Other Supplementary Studies* (Philadelphia: F.A. Davis).

Garber, M. (1992) *Vested Interests: Cross-Dressing and Cultural Anxiety* (New York: Harper Perennial).

Gattari, P., L. Spizzichino, C. Valenzi, M. Zaccarelli, and G. Rezza (1992) "Behavioural Patterns and HIV Infection among Drug Using Transvestites Practicing Prostitution in Rome," *AIDS Care*, 4:83–87.

Goihman S., A. Ferreira, S. Santos, and J.L. Grandi (1994) "Silicone Application as a Risk Factor for HIV Infection," *X International Conference on AIDS*, Yokohama, August 7–12.

Grandi J.L., A.C. Ferreira, and A. Kalichman (1993) "HIV and Syphilis Infection among Transvestites in São Paulo City," *IX International Conference on AIDS*, Berlin, June 6–11.

Hirschfeld, M. (1910) *Die Transvestiten: Eine Untersuchung über den Erotischen Verkleidungstrieb mit Anfanfreichem Casuistischen und Historischen Material* (Leipzig: Max Spohr).

Inciardi, J.A. and H.L. Surratt (1995) "The Use of the Female Condom for Anal Sex," *III National Conference of Transvestites and the Liberated*, Rio de Janeiro, Brazil, June 13–16.

Inciardi, J.A. and H.L. Surratt (1996) "The Female Condom and the Prevention of AIDS," *International Forum on the Prevention of Drug Use and AIDS*, Institute for the Development of the Amazon, Belem, Brazil, April 19.

Kulick, D. (1998) *Travesti: Sex, Gender and Culture among Brazilian Transgendered Prostitutes* (Chicago: University of Chicago Press).

Linger, D.T. (1992) *Dangerous Encounters: Meaning of Violence in a Brazilian City* (Stanford, CA: Stanford University Press).

Lukianowicz, N. (1959) "Survey of Various Aspects of Transvestism in Light of Our Present Knowledge," *Journal of Nervous and Mental Disease*, 128: 36–64.

Manchete (1997) 46 (15 February).

Nanda, S. (1985) "The Hijras of India: Cultural and Individual Dimensions of an Institutionalized Third Gender Role," *Journal of Homosexuality*, 11: 35–54.

Parker, R.G. (1989) "Youth, Identity, and Homosexuality: The Changing Shape of Sexual Life in Brazil," *Journal of Homosexuality*, 17: 269–289.

Parker, R. (1999) *Beneath the Equator* (New York: Routledge).

Prince, V. and P.M. Bentler (1972) "Survey of 504 Cases of Transvestism," *Psychological Reports*, 31:903–917.

Scheper-Hughes, N. (1992) *Death Without Weeping: The Violence of Everyday Life in Brazil* (Berkeley: University of California Press).

Stoller, R.J. (1971) "The Term 'Transvestism,'" *Archives of General Psychiatry*, 24:230–237.

Suleiman J., G. Suleiman, and G.P.A. Ayroza (1989) "Seroprevalence of HIV among Transvestites in the City of São Paulo," *V International Conference on AIDS*, Montreal, June 4–9.

Taylor, E. (1994) *Rio de Janeiro* (Boston: Houghton Mifflin).

Telles, P.R., H.L. Surratt, and J.A. Inciardi (1996) "Assessing the Regional Distribution of HIV Prevalence among Drug Users in Rio de Janeiro," *XI International Conference on AIDS,* Vancouver, July 7–12.

Chapter 7

Adams, I., R. Martins, M. Campos and J. Paiva (1994) "The Ammor Population," *10th International Conference on AIDS,* Yokohama.

Almeida, M.(1978) "Contrabucion al Estudio de la Historia Natural de la Dependencia a la Pasta Basica de Cocaina," *Revista de Neuro-Psiquiatria,* 41:44–45.

Archambault, C. (1989) "Rio's Shaky Shantytowns," *IRDC Reports,* (April):18–19.

Barker, G.(1992) "More Than a Minor Problem," *Institute of the Americas Hemisfile,* 3 (January):6.

Brookes, S. (1991) "Life on Rio's Mean Streets," *Insight,* 5, (August 5):12–19.

Burns, E.(1980) *A History of Brazil* (New York: Columbia University Press).

Butterworth, D. and J.K. Chance (1981) *Latin American Urbanization* (Cambridge: Cambridge University Press).

Campos, R., C. Antunes, M. Jeronymo, M. Raffaelli, A. Payne-Merritt, N.Halsey, and D. Greco (1992) "Comparison of Behavioral Risks for HIV Infection among Sub-Groups of Brazilian Street Youth," *8th International Conference on AIDS,* Amsterdam.

Campos,R., M. Greco, W. Ude, A. Machado, M. Raffaelli, M. Campos and D. Greco (1994) "Female Street Youths: Social Factors Associated to Behavioral Risks for HIV Infection," *10th International Conference on AIDS,* Yokohama.

Campos, R., M. Raffaelli, W. Ude, M. Greco, A. Ruff, J. Rolf, C. Antunes, N. Halsey and D. Greco (1994) "Social Networks and Daily Activities of Street Youth in Belo Horizonte, Brazil," *Child Development,* 65:319–330.

Carlini, E.A. and B. Carlini-Cotrim (1993) "Illicit Use of Psychotropic Drugs among Brazilian Students: 1987 and 1989 Surveys, in *Brasil"—United States Binational Research,* eds. M.G. Monteiro and J.A. Inciardi, 151–163 (São Paulo: CEBRID).

Carlini-Cotrim, B. and E.A. Carlini (1988) "The Use of Solvents and Other Drugs among Children and Adolescents from a Low Socio-Economic Background: A Study in São Paulo, Brazil," *International Journal of the Addictions,* 23:1145–1156.

De Paula, I. (1992) "Drugs Used by 100 Percent of Street Children," *Brasília Correio Braziliense* 10(May):2.

Dewees, A. and S.J. Klees (1995) "Social Movements and the Transformation of National Policy: Street and Working Children in Brazil," *Comparative Education Review,* 39(1):76–100.

Dimenstein, G. (1991) *Brazil: War on Children* (London: Latin American Bureau).

Dos Passos, J. (1963) *"Brazil on the Move* (New York: Paragon House).

Eisenstein, E. (1993) "Street Youth: Social Imbalance and Health Risks," *Journal of Paediatrics and Child Health,* 29(suppl 1):S46-S49.

Eisenstein, E. (1994) "Access to Health Services Specially [Sic] in Relation to Street Children and Drugs," Presented at Conference on Street Children and Psychoactive Substances, Geneva, Switzerland.

Eisenstein, E., and M.T. De Aquino,(1992) "Street Children and Drugs Rio de Janeiro: Núcleo de Estudos e Pesquisas em Atenção ao Uso de Drogas," Unpublished manuscript.

Ellison, K. (1994)"Rio's Tough Street Kids Still Live in Fear," *Miami Herald* (July 28):12A

Facts on File. (1996) "Officer Convicted in Massacre of Youths," *Facts on File, 56,* (May 9):328–329.

Firebaugh, G. (1979) "Structural Determinants of Urbanization in Asia and Latin America," *American Sociological Review,* 44:199–215.

Freyre, G. (1986) *The Mansions and the Shanties* (Berkeley: University of California Press).

Guillermoprieto, A. (1990) *Samba* (New York: Alfred A. Knopf).

Gunther, J. (1966) *Inside South America* (New York: Harper and Row).

International Child Resource Institute (1996) *Brazil Street Children Bulletin* (Fall):1–2.

Jeri, F.R. (1984) "Coca-Paste Smoking in Some Latin American Countries: A Severe and Unabated Form of Addiction" *Bulletin on Narcotics* (April-June):15–31.

Jeri, F.R., C. Sanchez, and T. Del Pozo (1976) "Consumo de Drogal PeligRosas por Miembros Familiares de la Fuerza Armada y Fuerza Policial Peruana," *Revista de la Sanidad de las Fuerzas Policiales,* 37:104–112.

Kirsch, H., ed. (1995) *Drug Lessons and Education Programs in Developing Countries* (New Brunswick, NJ: Transaction Publishers).

Larmer, B. (1992) "Dead End Kid," *Newsweek,* 119 *(May 25):38–41.*

Loveman, B. (1991) "Latin America Faces Public Enemy No. 1," *Hemisfile* 2(July): 6–8.

Lusk, M.W. (1989) "Street Children Programs in Latin America," *Journal of Sociology and Social Welfare,* 16:55–77.

Martins, J.P.S. (1992) "Brazilian Police Go after Street Children," *Latinamerica Press* (April 16):7.

Michaels, M. (1993) "Rio's Dead End Kids," *Time,* 142 (August 9):36–37.

Pinto, J.A., A. Ruff, J.V. Paiva, C.M. Antunes, I. Adams, N. Halsey, and D. Greco (1992) "Comparative Assessment of Risk Behavior and Seroprevalence of HIV–1 among Homeless and Underprivileged Youth in Belo Horizonte, Brazil," Presented at 8th International Conference on AIDS, Amsterdam, The Netherlands.

Raffaelli, M., P. Merritt, R. Campos, E. Siqueira, W. Ude, M. Greco, D. Greco, and N. Halsey (1992) "Correlates of Condom Use among Street Youth in Belo Horizonte, Brazil," *Presented at the 8th International Conference on AIDS,* Amsterdam, The Netherlands.

Rambali, P. (1993) *In the Cities and Jungles of Brazil* (New York: Henry Holt).

Raphael, A., and J. Berkman (1992) "Children Without a Future," *Brazil Network* (September):1–35.

Rizzini, I. and M.W. Lusk, (1995) "Children in the Streets: Latin America's Lost Generation," *Children and Youth Services Review,* 17(3):391–400.

Saum, C.A., and J.A. Inciardi (1997) "Rohypnol Misuse in the United States," *Substance Use and Misuse,* 32:723–731.

Scheper-Hughes, N., and D. Hoffman (1994) "Kids out of Place," *NACLA Report on the Americas* 27, (May/June):16–23.

Siqueira, E., P. Merritt, W. Ude, R. Campos, M. Greco, M. Raffaelli, N. Halsey, and D. Greco, (1992) "HIV Outreach Communication Intervention for Brazilian Street Youth," Presented at 8th International Conference on AIDS, Amsterdam, The Netherlands.

Thomas, J.J. (1995) *Surviving the City: The Urban Informal Sector in Latin America* (London: Pluto Press).

Ude, W., A. Payne, C. Antunes, E. Holt, M. Raffaelli, Z. Ottone, J. Rolf, J. Pinto, J. Paiva, R. Campos, M. Greco, E. Siqueira, D. Greco, A. Ruff, and N. Halsey, (1991) "A Comparison of Three Methods of Obtaining Information from Street Youths Regarding HIV Risk Behaviors," Presented at 7th International Conference on AIDS, Florence, Italy.

United Nations Children's Fund (1996a) *The State of the World's Children: 1996* (Geneva: UNICEF).

United Nations Children's Fund (1996b) *Country Profile: Brazil* (Geneva: UNICEF).

Van Buuren, N. and C.A. Bezerra (1992) "The Need to Open a Discussion about a Public Secret," Presented at 8th International Conference on AIDS, Amsterdam, The Netherlands.

Vasconcelos, A. (1990) *SOS Meninas*, Recife, (Brazil: Casa de Passagem).

Wiik, F.B., A. Filgueiras, and M.L. CASTRO,(1989) "Street Teenagers and an AIDS Prevention Program in Brazil," Presented at 5th International Conference on AIDS, Montreal, Canada.

Epilogue

Alexandrino, M. (1991) "AIDS: Santos Iniciará Estudo com Viciados," *O Globo* (March 10):46.

Barbosa de Carvalho, H., F. Mesquita, E. Massad, R.C. Bueno, G.T. Lopes, M.A. Ruiz, and M.N. Burattini (1996) "HIV and Infections of Similar Transmission Patterns in a Drug Injectors Community of Santos, Brazil," *Journal of Acquired Immune Deficiency Syndromes and Human Retrovirology*, 12:84–92.

Brazilian Ministry of Health (1991) *Normas e Procedimentos na Abordagem do Abuso de Drogas* (Brasília: Secretaria Nacional de Assistência à Saúde).

Brazilian Ministry of Health (1997a) *Boletim Epidemiológico de AIDS*, X, no. 3 (June-August).

Brazilian Ministry of Health (1997b) *Indicadores: Morbidade*, November.

Diário Oficial (1997) *Assessoria Técnico-Legislativa*, September 17.

Federal Narcotics Council (1994) "Ata da 4ª Reunião Ordinária," August 1.

Flowers, Nancy M. (1988) "The Spread of AIDS in Rural Brazil," in R. Kulstad (ed.), *AIDS 1988* (Washington, DC: American Association for the Advancement of Science).

Inciardi, J.A. and L.D. Harrison (1999) "The Concept of Harm Reduction," in J.A. Inciardi and L.D. Harrison (eds.), *Harm Reduction: National and International Perspectives* (Thousand Oaks, CA: Sage Publications).

Inciardi, J.A., H.L. Surratt, and P.R. Telles (1998) "HIV/AIDS Harm Reduction Through Community Outreach and Intervention in Rio de Janeiro, Brazil," *International Conference on the Reduction of Drug Related Harm*, São Paulo, Brazil, March 15–19.

Inciardi, J.A., H.L. Surratt, P.R. Telles, C.B. McCoy, H.V. McCoy, and N.L. Weatherby (1996) "Risks for HIV–1 Infection and Seropositivity Rates among Cocaine Users in Rio de Janeiro, Brazil," *XI International Conference on AIDS*, Vancouver, British Columbia, July 7–12.

Jornal do Brasil (1994) "Incidência da AIDS é Maior Entre Viciados," August 2, p. 7.

Laranjeira, R. and I. Pinsky (1996) "O Crack e a Prefeitura," *O Estado de São Paulo*, September 16.

Lima, E.S., F.I. Bastos, P.R. Telles, and T.P. Ward (1992) "Injecting Drug Users and the Spread of HIV in Brazil," *AIDS & Public Policy Journal*, 7:170–174.

O Estado de São Paulo (1995) "Apreendido Material Anti-AIDS em Santos," December 18.

O Estado de São Paulo (1996a) "Deputado Quer Mudar Lei Sobre Drogas," January 23.

O Estado de São Paulo (1996b) "Seringas Serão Distribuídas para Conter AIDS," June 24.

Parker, R.G. (1992) "AIDS Education and Health Promotion in Brazil: Lessons from the Past and Prospects for the Future," in J. Sepulveda, H. Fineberg, and J. Mann (eds.), *AIDS: Prevention Through Education—A World View* (Oxford: Oxford University Press).

Segatto, C. (1997) "SP Distribuirá Seringas a Consumidores de Drogas," *O Estado de São Paulo*, September 19.

Silva, S.C. (1997) "Governo Quer Distribuir Seringa a Viciados," *O Estado de São Paulo*, March 19.

State Council on AIDS Issues (1994) "Projeto de Prevenção ao Abuso de Drogas, DST e AIDS no Ministério da Saúde," *News Brief*, December 8.

State Secretary of Health STD/AIDS Division (1995) "Recomendações Gerais aos Profissionais de Saúde da Rede Pública Estadual para a Prevenção da Infecção pelo HIV entre Usuários de Drogas Injetáveis," *Position paper*, May.

State Secretary of Health STD/AIDS Division (1997) *Boletim Epidemiológico Sobre AIDS*, January/February/March.

Surratt, H.L., W.M. Wechsberg, L. Cottler, C.G. Leukefeld, H. Klein, and D. Desmond (1998) "Acceptability of the Female Condom among Women at Risk for HIV Infection," *American Behavioral Scientist*, 41(8):1157–1170.

Telles, P.R. (1997) *Projeto Redução de Danos Entre Usuários de Drogas Injetáveis no Rio de Janeiro: Relatório de Evolução*, June.

Telles, P.R. (1999) "Preventing HIV/AIDS and Other Sexually Transmitted Diseases among Injecting Drug Users in Rio de Janeiro," *International Journal of Drug Policy*, 10:365–373.

Telles, P.R., F.I. Bastos, F. Mesquita, R. Stall, N. Hearst, and R. Bueno (1994) "Assessing Risk Behaviors and HIV Seroprevalence among IDUs in Two Major Ports of South America," *X International Conference on AIDS*, Yokohama, August 7–12.

Telles, P.R., M. Cruz, W. Bastos Jr., C. Sampaio, R. Mazzuia, and L. Guanabara (1998) "Managing HIV Diffusion among Injecting Drug Users in Rio de Janeiro, Brazil," *International Conference on Drug-Related Harm*, São Paulo, March 15–19.

Tomaleza, J. (1996) "Sorocaba Terá Clínica Pública para Recuperação de Viciados," *O Estado de São Paulo*, December 26.

Watters, J.K. and P. Biernacki (1989) "Targeted Sampling: Options for theStudy of Hidden Populations." *Social Problems,* 36:416–430.

World Health Organization (1993) "An International Comparative Study of HIV Prevalence and Risk Behavior among Drug Injectors in 13 cities," *Bulletin on Narcotics,* 45:19–46.

Appendix B

Burdick, J. (1995) "Brazil's Black Consciousness Movement," in K. Danaher and M. Shellenberger (eds.), *Fighting for the Soul of Brazil,* (New York: Monthly Review Press).

Degler, C.N. (1971) *Neither Black nor White: Slavery and Race Relations in Brazil and the United States* (New York: Macmillan).

Ellison, K. (1995) "Brazil's Blacks, Building Pride, Invoke the Legend of Rebel Warrior Zumbi," *Miami Herald,* November 19:1A.

Goering, L. (1994) "Brazilian Harmony among Races Not as Strong As it Seems," *Philadelphia Inquirer,* December 26:A12.

Haberly, D.T. (1995) "Three Sad Races," in G. Harvey Summ (ed.), *Brazilian Mosaic: Portraits of a Diverse People and Culture,* (Wilmington, DE: Scholarly Resources).

Hanchard, M.G. (1994) *Orpheus and Power: The Movimento Negro of Rio de Janeiro and São Paulo, Brazil, 1945–1988* (Princeton, NJ: Princeton University Press).

Harris, M.(1970) "Referential Ambiguity in the Calculus of Brazilian Racial Identity," *Southwestern Journal of Anthropology,* 27:1–14.

Harris, M., J. Consorte, J. Lang, and B. Byrne (1993) "Who Are the Whites?: Imposed Census Categories and the Racial Demography of Brazil," *Social Forces,* 72:451–462.

Harrison, P.A. (1995) "Behaving Brazilian," in G. Harvey Summ (ed.), *Brazilian Mosaic: Portraits of a Diverse People and Culture,* (Wilmington, DE: Scholarly Resources).

Hasenbalg, C.(1985) "Race and Socioeconomic Inequalities in Brazil," in P. Fontaine (ed.), *Race, Class, and Power in Brazil,* (Los Angeles: University of California Press).

Hasenbalg, C. and S. Huntington (1982) "Brazilian Racial Democracy: Reality or Myth?" *Humboldt Journal of Social Relations,* 10:129–142.

Skidmore, T.E. (1972) "Toward a Comparative Analysis of Race Relations since Abolition in Brazil and the United States," *Latin American Studies,* 4:1–28.

Wagley, C. (1952) *Race and Class in Rural Brazil* (New York: Columbia University Press).

Winant, H. (1994) *Racial Conditions: Politics, Theory, Comparisons* (Minneapolis: University of Minnesota Press).

Wood, C.H. and J.A. Magno de Carvalho (1988) *The Demography of Inequality in Brazil* (Cambridge: Cambridge University Press).

Index

About the Authors

James A. Inciardi, Ph.D. is the Director of the Center for Drug and Alcohol Studies at the University of Delaware; a professor in the Department of Sociology and Criminal Justice at Delaware; and a guest professor in the Department of Psychiatry at the Federal University of Rio Grande do Sul in Porto Alegre, Brazil, and was the Principal Investigator of the Brazil-based HIV/AIDS prevention/intervention project.

Hilary L. Surratt, M.A. is an Associate Scientist in the Center for Drug and Alcohol Studies at the University of Delaware, and was the Co-Principal Investigator and Project Director of the Brazil-based HIV/AIDS prevention/intervention project.

Paulo R. Telles, M.D., Ph.D. is a Senior Researcher in the Nucleo de Estudos e Pesquisas em Atenção ao Uso de Drogas at the State University of Rio de Janeiro, and was the Scientific Director of the Brazil-based HIV/AIDS prevention/intervention project.